Speech and Language Therapists and Mental Capacity

The use of general descriptive names, registered names, trademarks, etc. in this publication does not imply, even in the absence of a specific statement, that such names are exempt from the relevant protective laws and regulations and therefore free for general use.

British Library Cataloguing in Publication Data
A catalogue record for this book is available from the British Library

Cover design: Jim Wilkie
Cover image : Nicola Markovic used under license from Shutterstock.com
Project management, typesetting and design: J&R Publishing Services Ltd, Guildford, Surrey, UK; www.jr-publishingservices.co.uk

Disclaimer

It is important to note that the information contained in this book provides only an overview of the legal requirements for managing decision-making capacity and other aspects outlined in the Mental Capacity Act, 2005, within England and Wales, the Adults with Incapacity (Scotland) Act 2000 and the Mental Capacity Act (Northern Ireland) 2016. Readers should ensure they have read and understood the relevant legal framework for their location and refer to this when planning and conducting capacity assessments or any other practice related to this. Reliance should not be placed on the opinions set out in this book and readers must take their own legal advice. The authors cannot take any responsibility for readers' practice that is not consistent with the law.

Printed and bound by CPI Group (UK) Ltd, Croydon, CR0 4YY

Speech and Language Therapists and Mental Capacity

A training resource for adult services

Isla Jones and Anna Volkmer
(Editors)

J&R Press Ltd

"Involving people in decisions about their care is intrinsic to the principles of the MCA and should be evident in every care and support plan."
   SCIE website accessed 25 March 2018

https://www.scie.org.uk/mca/practice/care-planning/person-centred-care

Contents

Contributors

Dr Daniel J Bailey, MA FRCP, Consultant Physician/Geriatrician, Department of Clinical Gerontology, King College Hospital

Karen Bamford[1], Clinical Lead Speech and Language Therapist, Learning Disabilities Services, Birmingham Community Healthcare Trust, UK

Rachel Daly, DN, RN, BIA, MSc, BA (Hons), Queens Nurse

James Godber, Mental Capacity Act Practitioner/Speech and Language Therapist based in Adult Safeguarding Team at St George's University Hospitals NHS Foundation Trust

Dr Mark Jayes, Research Fellow in Communication Disability, Manchester Metropolitan University

Isla Jones, Specialist Speech and Language Therapist Elderly Care/Geriatrics

Anna Robinson, Speech and Language Therapist

Dr Lucy Series, Wellcome Research Fellow and Lecturer in Law, School of Law and Politics, Cardiff University

Anna Volkmer, Highly Specialist Speech and Language Therapist, NIHR Doctoral Research Fellow, University College London

---

1 Deceased

Acknowledgements

We would like to acknowledge Dr Lucy Series, Dr Dan Bailey, James Godber, Rachel Daly, Dr Mark Jayes and Anna Robinson for their commitment to this project. Particular thanks to Karen Bamford and all the SLTs in her team who continued the capacity conversation in the *Bulletin* magazine and then wrote numerous case examples for this book. They have made contributions without which this book would not be possible.

I would also like to thank all those who 'believe in the writing' on this resource including Rachael Wilkie, Dr Suzanne Beeke and all my colleagues. I couldn't do this without my family; both for their emotional support (James Morgan and Helen Pridham) and their thorough proofreading skills (Helen Pridham, Paula Volkmer, Tessa Volkmer). And, of course, the cheering squad- Kate McCabe-Simon. *(Anna Volkmer)*

I would like to acknowledge Lorna Jacques and Paul Jones for their proofreading and helpful comments. Also, my colleagues and clinical lead Lynne Clark for their insights, questions and encouragement. Finally, Scott Reeve for his endless support and patience. *(Isla Jones)*

Foreword

Mental capacity legislation is concerned with that most fundamental expression of our identity: making decisions about our own lives. The Adults with Incapacity (Scotland) Act 2000 and the Mental Capacity Act 2005 of England and Wales were considered 'visionary' pieces of legislation for their time.[2] The Mental Capacity Act (Northern Ireland) 2016 is the world's first example of 'fusion' legislation, bringing together mental health laws with guardianship legislation and using the concept of 'mental capacity' for both.

The purpose of mental capacity legislation is often described as to 'empower and protect' people who may have difficulty making decisions. Yet many people are routinely excluded from what is increasingly recognized as a 'right' to make decisions about their own lives because of problems communicating. This much-needed book draws attention to the role that speech and language therapists can play in supporting this right.

Speech and language therapists can play a vital role in helping to secure and broaden the rights of people with communication impairments to make decisions for themselves. Speech and language therapists can play a pivotal role in building and developing a person's own communication skills, but equally – if not more important – is their help in challenging the environments and attitudes that inhibit good communication for people with diverse needs.

Under UK capacity laws, a person who is assessed as unable to understand the information relevant to the decision, to retain that information long enough to make a decision, to use and weigh or 'appreciate' this information, or to communicate their decision as others, is considered to lack the 'mental capacity' to make this decision for themselves. Those assessing mental capacity must help the person to make the decision for themselves before concluding that they lack mental capacity. If a person is assessed as lacking mental capacity, then others can make decisions in their 'best interests' (in England, Wales, and Northern Ireland) or for their 'benefit' (in Scotland). Those making substitute decisions have a legal obligation to consider the subjective views of the person, past and present, and to help them to participate in the decision as fully as possible.

There is a temptation to view 'mental capacity' as only being about the abilities of the person. Speech and language therapists will know better than

---

2   House of Lords Select Committee on the Mental Capacity Act 2005, *Mental Capacity Act 2005: Post-legislative scrutiny* (HL Paper 139, 2014).

this – they will be aware that the skills of the assessor, and the environmental context of the assessment, are just as relevant. Those assessing a person must be able to communicate the relevant information as effectively as they can to that individual, to provide support to the person in making the decision, and to understand the person's own perspective as fully as they can. It is troubling to think of how many people will have lost the right to make decisions of great importance to them because they were assessed by an individual who did not have the time, skills, or resources to communicate effectively with them. As a profession, speech and language therapists can play an important role in enhancing the skills of assessors and the context of assessment across other professions, as well as undertaking assessments themselves.

This book by Anna Volkmer and Isla Jones is timely. The importance of supporting an individual to make a decision for themselves has increased following the adoption by the United Nations of the Convention on the Rights of Persons with Disabilities (CRPD) in 2006, which was ratified by the UK in 2009. Article 12 of the CRPD, the right to equal recognition before the law, says that states must ensure that disabled people have access to the supports they need in exercising legal capacity. It says that disabled people must be able to enjoy legal capacity (making legal decisions) on an equal basis with others, and that the goal of support must be to give expression to the person's 'will and preferences'. The Committee is highly critical of the two core concepts of the MCA – it views 'mental capacity' as a discriminatory test, and 'best interests' as an outdated paternalistic approach that violates human rights.[3] The Committee states that supported decision may take diverse forms, and that assistance with communication, and the recognition of 'diverse, non-conventional methods of communication' may be central to realising this right for some. The Committee has urged the UK to speed up research and develop good practices in supported decision making.[4]

Although it has not gone as far as the Committee's radical proposals to abolish all forms of substitute decision making, the Law Commission has recommended that the Mental Capacity Act 2005 be amended to place *more* emphasis on the person's wishes, feelings, values and beliefs[5], and the

3 Committee on the Rights of Persons with Disabilities, *General Comment No 1 (2014) Article 12: Equal recognition before the law* (19 May 2014, CRPD/C/GC/1, 2014).

4 Committee on the Rights of Persons with Disabilities, *Concluding Observations on the United Kingdom* (29 August 2017, UN Doc CRPD/C/GBR/CO/1, 2017).

5 Law Commission, *Mental Capacity and Deprivation of Liberty* (Law Com No 372, 2017).

government has accepted this recommendation.[6] The Scottish Government is undertaking a review of the Adults with Incapacity (Scotland) Act 2000 in view of the CRPD.[7] The government has also instructed the National Institute for Clinical Excellence to prepare guidelines on mental capacity and supported decision making, and these are under preparation.[8] Anna Volkmer has played a role in developing these guidelines, and they emphasize the important role played by speech and language therapists in supporting decision making and improving the context of mental capacity assessments.

Our current laws are most probably not compliant with the CRPD, but front-line professionals must do the best they can to maximize rights to decision making under existing domestic laws. What role can speech and language professionals play, as a profession, in helping the UK to move forward in protecting rights to decide? Clearly, speech and language professionals can apply their knowledge of good communication when assessing mental capacity in their own clinical practice. But their role can be much broader than this. As a profession, speech and language therapists can raise awareness among other colleagues – including in health and social care, but also further afield such as law and finance – of the role that communication plays in supporting decision making. They can offer training, guidance and consultancy to public and private sector services to help them maximize the opportunities for good communication to take place in the diverse contexts in which we make key decisions about our lives, from the hospital bed, care home or family home, to banks and solicitors' offices.

Speech and language therapists can also champion the role that communication plays in supporting decision making through acting as experts in the Court of Protection. At the moment, there is a tendency to view psychiatrists and other medical professionals as 'the experts' on assessing mental capacity, but in practice they may lack expertise in facilitating good communication. In a recent court case a judge rejected an assessment by a psychiatrist that a man with learning disabilities lacked mental capacity as they had used no 'tangible techniques' to support his decision making. Instead, they

---

6 HM Government, *Final Government Response to the Law Commission's Review of Deprivation of Liberty Safeguards and Mental Capacity* (Department of Health and Social Care written statement, 14 March 2018, 2018).

7 Scottish Government, *Adults with Incapacity (Scotland) Act 2000 Proposals for Reform* (2018).

8 National Institute for Clinical Excellence, 'Decision making and mental capacity' (In development GID-NG10009, expected publication date: 29 May 2018) < https://www.nice.org.uk/guidance/indevelopment/gid-ng10009> [accessed 27 March 2018].

preferred the evidence of a social worker who spent three days with the man, getting to know him in his home and using pictorial aids to find out what his thoughts and feelings were about the options available, and who concluded that he had mental capacity.[9] Speech and language therapists have a wealth of knowledge of these kinds of tangible techniques.

This book provides an excellent foundation for training and guidance for speech and language therapists who are keen to apply these principles in their own clinical practice, and to promote their role more widely in supporting people's rights to make decisions about their lives. It covers a range of settings and contexts and provides an excellent overview of the relevant law and policy. I look forward to seeing how speech and language therapists will contribute to growing awareness of the importance of good communication in supporting rights to decide, and working with others to make these rights a reality.

Dr Lucy Series, School of Law and Politics, Cardiff University

28 March 2018

---

9 *LBX v K, L, M* [2013] EWHC 3230 (Fam).

1 The mental capacity legislation across England and Wales, Scotland and Northern Ireland: Relevance to healthcare

Dan Bailey

Introduction

Mental capacity legislation has been in place, in the UK, for almost 20 years. Mental capacity issues are common in healthcare. It is a complex subject that can leave some professionals anxious about putting it into practice. This chapter looks at the importance of mental capacity in a societal context before moving on to define this concept. The relevance of mental capacity is explained in relation to healthcare, and the distinctions made between mental capacity in physical and mental health. The final part of this chapter compares the three different pieces of UK mental capacity legislation across England and Wales, Scotland and Northern Ireland. Other aspects of mental capacity law (e.g., assessment of best interests and Deprivation of Liberty Safeguards) and mental health law are beyond the scope of this chapter. The chapter concludes with a brief discussion of the case for reforming the current law.

Decisions and society

Our society places high value on the ability and freedom of an individual to shape the course of their own life. We grow up expecting to take decisions that affect the direction of our lives, based on the belief that we have the best knowledge and understanding of our internal value and judgement systems to make such choices. We feel, therefore, that only we can judge what is best for us. If this ability is taken away from us we feel thwarted and frustrated.

Our capacity for free and independent action, on the basis of thoughts and decisions, is known as 'autonomy', literally the ability of self-rule (Hope, 2004, p. 65). There are limits, however, on our ability to do exactly as we might choose. Our actions can be restricted by the law, by morality, and by society, with the aim of protecting both individuals and society from the unacceptable consequences of unwise or dangerous decisions. We accept these constraints, even though we value protection of the right to individual autonomy.

Previously, healthcare was an area in which we accepted limits on the autonomous control of our lives. The culture of "Doctor knows best …" meant that service users unquestioningly followed the decisions made by their doctor. Such beneficent paternalism has been rejected within bioethics, with service-user autonomy and self-determination now understood as a basic human right (Brazier & Cave, 2007, p. 99). We must respect service user decisions and choices, positioning ourselves as partners in promoting good health (Brazier & Cave, 2007, p. 5), and helping service users to make their own decisions about treatment. This is not easy, as we may have to respect decisions that objectively appear to be wrong (Hope, 2004, p. 65), whilst experiencing potential moral and emotional distress (Richardson, 2013, p. 87).

Richardson (2013, p. 89) reminds us that the ability to make a decision for oneself is an integral part of our legal framework. She explains that the law sets out the standards which allow us to determine whether a decision is legally effective or not. If it is, then it will be respected. People with mental capacity to make a decision will have legal capacity for that decision. People lacking mental capacity to make a decision may not have their choice for that decision followed. Decisions made for other people have to be regulated. In the UK mental capacity legislation covers this.

Mental capacity

The term 'mental capacity' is synonymous with the terms 'competence' and 'decision making capacity'. The Mental Capacity Act 2005 Code of Practice (MCA 2005 Code of Practice, 2007, p. 41) defines it as, "…the ability to make a decision". It states that a person can be said to have capacity if they can make that decision for themselves. The range of decisions that a person can make are, in theory, limitless, although I have already noted that some choices are prohibited by law even if the person has capacity to choose them.

Individual societies use different models to determine the threshold at which a person has capacity. These can be based on a person's status, e.g., that people under a certain age do not have capacity to make decisions. They can also be based on the person's functional ability in decision making (Jackson, 2006, p. 192). In the UK both approaches are employed: children under the age of 18 are presumed to lack capacity unless they can prove they have it; and adults are presumed to have capacity unless it can be proven that they lack it (Jackson, 2006, p. 193). It is rare, however, for people to be deemed to lack capacity to make all decisions, as it is not considered to be an 'all or nothing matter'. It admits of degrees and depends on the complexity of the decision to be made and the risks that are involved (Grisso & Applebaum, 1998, pp. 32-33).

Mental capacity and healthcare

Mental capacity is an important area in healthcare practice. It is part of the legal standard for valid consent, the others being voluntariness (i.e., being free from coercion), and understanding the nature of what is proposed (Jackson, 2006, p. 255). Any procedure carried out without valid consent is unlawful, so it is essential that we know whether service users have capacity to consent to treatment before we proceed with it. In addition to this, we have a duty to respect service user autonomy (Hope, 2004, p. 5) and therefore need to know whether people have capacity to make decisions.

Mental capacity is decision-specific. It is meaningless to state that a person 'lacks capacity' (Ruck Keene et al., 2016, p. 2), except in a few circumstances, e.g., coma or profound cognitive impairment. Phrases such as this suggest that the person making the statement does not understand the nature of capacity assessment.

In order to make capacity assessments meaningful, we must be clear about the decision the person must make. The choices people are asked to make can be complex. It might be necessary to break down a complex decision into a series of smaller ones.

Healthcare presents people with lots of decisions and choices. Healthcare professionals are often alerted to a potential lack of capacity when a person makes a decision that appears to be irrational or unwise (Jackson, 2006, p. 193). This is in spite of the central prominence of service user autonomy and self-determination. This approach may, in fact, miss a large number of people who assent to treatment but still lack capacity to consent to it (Raymont et al., 2004).

We have to assess a person's capacity for every decision that they make. UK legislation has different approaches towards the assessment of capacity.

In England and Wales this is set out in the Mental Capacity Act (MCA, 2005). Other jurisdictions are discussed and compared to the MCA later in this chapter. Before doing so, it is worth noting that a legal distinction is made between decisions related to physical health and those related to mental health. UK law mostly has separate statutes covering these two types of decisions. This leads to different approaches towards people who are unable to make decisions about treatment for mental and physical illness, and can lead to the compulsion of people for treatment of the former. There is sufficient material on the difference between the Mental Health Act and the MCA (2005) for an entirely separate book and further coverage of it is not possible here.

The Mental Capacity Act (2005) – England and Wales

Background and introduction

In 2005 the Mental Capacity Act (MCA) received Royal Assent. It came into force in 2007, providing a statutory framework for assessing decision-making capacity and for treating and managing people who lacked competence (MCA 2005 Code of Practice, 2007, p. 1). It was designed to assist and support people who might lack capacity and to protect these people from being overly restricted or controlled by other people (Department for Constitutional Affairs, 2007, p. 15 [Para 1.4]). It superseded common law cases that dealt with these areas.

The Act covers people aged 16 and over in England and Wales (MCA, 2005, s.2(5)). It applies to situations where a person who might lack capacity needs to make a decision. The range of decisions is not limited to healthcare, but covers day-to day- choices as well (MCA 2005 Code of Practice, 2007, p. 16). The Act is clear that it does not cover decisions related to family relationships, mental health act matters, voting rights, and unlawful killing or assisted suicide. Decisions in these areas can never be made on behalf of an individual and actions related to them cannot be carried out by any person or body, even the Court of Protection (MCA 2005 Code of Practice, 2007, p. 16). The Court of Protection might be asked to decide whether someone has capacity to make a decision, but cannot then initiate a course of action in the person's best interests in relation to it (MCA 2005 Code of Practice, 2007, p. 16). Application of the Act is not limited to any specific location within the jurisdiction. This means that the Act applies to people in any setting, (e.g., a hospital, solicitor's office, a care home, or their own home); what matters is that the person faces making a decision - it is not limited by where they are going to make it.

Principles of the Act

Section 1 of the MCA (2005) sets out five core principles that apply to everyone covered by it:

1. A person must be assumed to have capacity unless it is established that he lacks capacity.

2. A person is not to be treated as unable to make a decision unless all practicable steps to help him to do so have been taken without success.

3. A person is not to be treated as unable to make a decision merely because he makes an unwise decision.

4. An act done, or decision made, under this Act for or on behalf of a person who lacks capacity must be done, or made, in his best interests.

5. Before the act is done, or the decision is made, regard must be had to whether the purpose for which it is needed can be as effectively achieved in a way that is less restrictive of the person's rights and freedom of action.

The principles apply to all sections of the Act, but have a key impact on the nature of the capacity assessment itself. It is useful to look at a couple of these in more detail

Proof of incapacity

People making decisions do not have to prove that they have capacity. It is up to the person assessing capacity to prove that a person lacks it. When assessing a person's capacity, we need to know what level of evidence is required to prove that they do not have it. The Act explains that the 'standard of proof' required is on the balance of probabilities (MCA, 2005, s.2(4)). This means that the assessor needs to have a reasonable belief that it is more likely than not that the person lacks capacity to make the decision in question (Ruck Keene et al., 2016, p. 3; MCA 2005 Code pf Practice, 2007, p. 56). Scrutiny of 'reasonable belief' would be required if there was a legal challenge to an assessment of capacity related to a decision. Neither the Act nor the Code of Practice detail how this might be demonstrated. In some ways, it is a matter for the Court to determine, but they will look at documentation, as well as oral evidence, to determine this. It seems sensible, therefore, to provide a detailed account of the information and evidence used to reach the conclusion about the person's capacity.

Requirement for practical assistance

We are required to do everything practical to help people make a decision for themselves (MCA 2005 Code of Practice, 2007, p. 22). In this way we are helping them to promote their autonomy. We need to ensure that we have provided the relevant information required. In addition to this, we need to be mindful of any conditions, diagnoses or impairments affecting communication that we can adjust for. Examples of these, from the Code of Practice (2007, p. 29), could include:

- Use of simple language/visual aids
- Nonverbal communication
- Use of an interpreter
- Use of a care worker, speech and language therapist (SLT), family member, or advocate that might be more familiar to the person.

Finally, we need to consider whether we have chosen the best time and location for the discussion, and whether there is something else we could do to help the person learn, or understand, or gain the ability to make the decision (Ruck Keene et al., 2016, p. 5).

Who can assess capacity and when should they do it?

There is a common misconception that only medical professionals, particularly psychiatrists, are able to assess capacity (Ruck Keene et al., 2016, p. 3). The Code of Practice (2007, p. 53) explains that, depending on the nature of the decision, any person can assess capacity, including:

- A care worker involved in day-to-day choices
- A healthcare professional proposing a treatment, examination, or a complex decision
- A solicitor who is instructed by a person to represent them.

The list is not exhaustive and the most appropriate person to undertake the assessment is likely to be:

- Someone directly concerned with the person when the decision needs to be made, which could include an SLT
- Someone who knows the person best
- The person intending to carry out the decision on behalf of the person if they lack capacity, e.g., a social worker if that person has to decide on a change of residence.

Sometimes a professional opinion is required for major or complex decisions. This can help inform the assessor, but it is still their responsibility to determine whether the person has capacity (Ruck Keene et al., 2016, p. 3).

As previously highlighted, it is important to consider the appropriate time of day to conduct a capacity assessment. It is also important to consider the timing of the assessment more broadly. A person may present with a temporary loss of capacity, e.g., delirium, which might resolve. It is vital to consider whether the decision can wait until this time and therefore an assessment of capacity could be delayed.

What is the MCA test for capacity?

The capacity test has two parts: functional and diagnostic. Use of the term 'diagnostic' does not only apply to a medical diagnosis. It applies to "... an impairment of the functioning of, the mind or brain" (MCA, 2005, s.2(1)). This can be either permanent or temporary (MCA, 2005, s.2(2)).

When conducting an assessment one must first establish if the person is "unable to make a decision for himself in relation to the matter" (MCA, 2005, s.2(1)). This is the functional test. If they cannot make a decision then one must establish whether this is "... because of an impairment of the functioning of, the mind or brain". If this second, diagnostic, test is satisfied then it can be said that the person lacks capacity to make that decision. Section 2(3) of the Act is clear that someone may not be judged as lacking capacity based on age, appearance, a condition, or aspects of behaviour. It does not go into further detail about this, leaving the Code of Practice to provide further explanation.

The ordering and wording of the test is important. If one starts by looking at the requirements of the diagnostic test (i.e., looking for an impairment of the functioning of, the mind or brain), then it is possible to discriminate against people with certain disorders (e.g., to assume that a person with depression lacks capacity to make a decision). To prevent this, it is imperative that we first establish the inability to make the decision. Use of the term, '**because of**' in the diagnostic test is key, as it asks us to consider whether the impairment of the functioning of the mind or brain is the cause behind the inability to make a decision (Ruck Keene et al., 2016, pp. 6-7).

The functional test

The MCA (2005) sets out the functional test in section 3(1), stating that, "A person is unable to make a decision for himself if he is unable:

  (a) To understand the information relevant to the decision

  (b) To retain that information

  (c) To use or weigh that information as part of the process of making the decision, or

  (d) To communicate his decision (whether by talking, using sign language or any other means)."

If the person is unable to do any one part of the test then they are unable to make the decision at hand. The following discussion examines this in a little more detail.

How much does the person have to understand?

In order to assess a person's understanding of a decision, we must first ensure that they have been given sufficient relevant information. This would include:

- The nature of the decision (MCA, 2005, Code of Practice, 2007, p. 46)
- Reasons why the decision is required
- Information on alternative choices (MCA, 2005, Code of Practice, 2007, p. 29)
- The implications of not making a decision at all (MCA, 2005, s.3).

The person does not have to understand every detail of what is explained to them, but must understand the salient factors (Ruck Keene et al., 2016, p. 7). The assessor must ensure that they do not expect too high a level of understanding (Ruck Keene et al., 2016, p. 8) and should decide what information is relevant and what the options might be. The person should be given the chance to understand the reality of the options (Ruck Keene et al., 2016, p. 8). This becomes more complex with abstract concepts and may be difficult if a person's understanding of such concepts is limited by their impairment. Over time, the courts have given indications as to the information that they feel is both relevant and irrelevant. Keene at al. have a good guide to this in the annex to their article (A Brief Guide to Carrying Out Capacity Assessments, 2016).

How long does a person have to retain the information for?

Capacity assessments have always involved an assessment of memory of the decision, which had the potential to disadvantage people with short-term memory problems. The MCA (2005) circumvents this in section 3(3) by specifying, "…the fact that a person is able to retain the information relevant to a decision for a short period only does not prevent him from being regarded as able to make the decision". The Code of Practice (p. 47) goes on to clarify that the person only needs to be able to hold the information long enough, "…to use it to make an effective decision". If, whilst being assessed, the person can retain the information for long enough to make a choice, then this is sufficient. There is no requirement for the person to retain memory of the information after the assessment.

How do we assess a person's ability to use or weigh information?

This is perhaps the most difficult and contentious part of the capacity test. The Code of Practice gives scant detail as to how to assess this. There has been a lot of case law that has examined this part of the test, some of which I will come to later.

In order to try to fully understand what is being tested, it is useful to look at work carried out in the United States by Grisso and Applebaum, to develop a standardized means of assessing decision-making abilities (Applebaum & Grisso, 1995, p. 106). They identified four legal standards to determine competence that are similar to those found in the MCA functional test. Two of these are similar to the standard of using and weighing information: the ability to appreciate a situation and its likely consequences, and the ability to manipulate information rationally (Applebaum & Grisso, 1995, p. 109). I will look at these now in an attempt to shed light on how we assess a person's ability to use and weigh information relevant to a decision.

In this model, the authors contend that the ability to appreciate information relevant to a choice is separate to simply understanding it (Grisso & Applebaum, 1998, p. 43). They hold that not having this skill refers to the inability of people to accept relevant disorders or potential treatment consequences for their own circumstances, due to either emotional or cognitive states (Grisso & Applebaum, 1998, p. 43). This might include an inability to acknowledge their illness or the consequences of their choices. If these emotional or cognitive states lead to beliefs relevant to the treatment decision that are substantially irrational, unrealistic, or a distortion of reality, then the person may have a lack of appreciation (Grisso & Applebaum, 1998, pp. 45, 47, 48). They are clear that this is more than just a disagreement with the physician's opinion (p. 45) but perhaps a failure to have insight into one's condition or situation. They recommend that an assessment of this ability would involve (p. 51):

- Enquiring into a person's beliefs underlying their reasoning

- Contextualizing these in terms of their physical and mental status

- Considering their religious and cultural background.

The ability to rationally manipulate information looks at the way a person uses and processes information relevant to a decision. It does not look at the rationality that informs the decision and does not consider the outcome either (Grisso & Applebaum, 1998, p. 53). Grisso and Applebaum identified a basic set of functions that are based on several problem-solving models (p. 54). They argue that a decision maker should be able to:

- Keep focus on the problem of selecting a course of action

- Take into account the range of available options during decision processing without narrowing their focus to one alternative, which would render the process meaningless

- Consider the consequences of the options and be able to imagine the consequences for 'his or her everyday life'

- Be able to think of the likelihood of the consequences occurring

- Weigh the desirability of the consequences, based on their subjective values

- Compare and work with the consequences, likelihood and desirability to reach a decision.

This functional description is useful but does not help us determine how we might assess them in a practical sense. The authors recommend the following (pp. 55-58):

- Encourage the person to think aloud through their decision

- Ascertain the degree to which they have considered the range of options and weighted the desirability of the consequences

- Establish whether the final choice flows logically from the person's view of the consequences.

None of the above is set out by English and Welsh law, but it makes for a useful start as to how to approach this part of the capacity test. It emphasizes the conversational nature of the capacity assessment and shows that it requires both a thorough discussion and a good understanding, or exploration, of the person's ideas, background, and beliefs. This means we have to think about our role as the assessor in the capacity assessment as well, because we will be the one deciding where the line between capacity and incapacity lies. MacDonald explained, "… the weight to be attached to that information in the decision making process is a matter for the decision maker" (Kings College Hospital NHS Foundation Trust and C and V, 2015, at para 38). Our ability to assess a person's usage and weighing of information will depend on our own belief systems. This is pertinent when a person makes a decision to refuse medical treatment considered to be necessary and appropriate by healthcare professionals, or when they continue to follow a risky course of action. The Courts (Kings College Hospital NHS Foundation Trust and C and V, 2015 at para 38) have explained that we must take care to try to avoid this:

> "…a person cannot be considered to be unable to use and weigh information simply on the basis that he or she has applied his or her own values or outlook to that information in making the decision in question and chosen to attach no weight to that information in the decision-making process."

This sets a high standard for this part of the assessment, and it is not clear how practicable it would be for assessors to provide such detailed analysis of a person's values and belief systems in order to establish that they are ignoring factors that a 'reasonable person' would take account of (Ruck Keene, 2017, p. 34). In Heart of England NHS Foundation Trust vs JB (2014, para. 7) the Court clarified that we must be careful to ensure that we carry out a detached and objective assessment that avoids the desire to protect the individual. We should not "...allow the tail of welfare to wag the dog of capacity".

In this part of the assessment we are going to have to show awareness for how a person processes information, how it fits into their belief systems, and how our own belief systems might bias our assessment of their decision making. As assessors, we will have to work hard during this conversation to try to understand diverse cultural and socio-economic differences. We may have to show respect for distinct idiosyncratic belief structures (Ruck Keene, 2017, p. 36) and will have to be prepared to delve deeply into service users' backgrounds and reasoning in order to give them a fair assessment.

It is worth making a final comment here about people who change their decision. A change of mind regarding a decision does not always mean that person has a problem using and weighing information related to it. It may be that, following the discussion, they have more time to think about the decision and change their choice. One should have concerns, however, about someone who changes their decision multiple times. This might indicate that they do have a problem using and weighing information. This could warrant a more detailed assessment and perhaps a second opinion.

How do we assess a person's ability to communicate a decision?

In the absence of clear inability to communicate, e.g., unconsciousness or profound communication impairment, but where there are apparent communication difficulties, there will need to be a detailed assessment of this and how to work around it. These are considered in further detail in Chapter 2.

The diagnostic test

After we have determined that a person cannot make a decision based on the criteria already described, the MCA (2005, s.2(1)) asks us to determine whether this inability is due to "... an impairment in the functioning of, the mind or brain". A person who does not satisfy the above criterion has capacity to make the decision at hand.

The Code of Practice (2007, p. 44) gives a nonexhaustive list of examples that might satisfy this criterion:

- Conditions associated with some forms of mental illness

- Dementia

- Significant learning disabilities

- The long-term effects of brain damage

- Physical or medical conditions that cause confusion, drowsiness or loss of consciousness

- Delirium

- Concussion following a head injury, and

- The symptoms of alcohol or drug use.

When considering this criterion, we must not draw conclusions about a person's capacity based on their behaviour, assumptions about their condition, or their appearance. We have to exercise care in assessing people with conditions that might have particular physical characteristics, e.g., cerebral palsy, or behavioural characteristics, e.g., intoxication from alcohol. We need to be sure that our assessment of their capacity only considers whether they are unable to undertake the parts of the functional test (related to a particular decision) and whether this inability is due to the impairment (MCA, 2005, Code of Practice, 2007, p. 43).

Documentation

The Act does not set out any provisions for documentation of capacity assessments. The Code of Practice suggests that professionals or paid care workers keep a record in their professional records. This might be the service user's clinical notes, or a care plan (MCA, 2005, Code of Practice, 2007, p. 63). In most healthcare settings, there will be a form to complete and to add to the service's notes. This should contain a detailed record of the discussion that took place and the evidence, or information, considered and used to reach the conclusion about the person's capacity to make the decision. The Care Quality Commission (CQC) is charged with checking that the Act is correctly implemented. One of the ways that they might do this is to look for records of assessments to show that capacity to consent to treatment and intervention was considered. Further discussion on implementation will be covered later in the book.

Discussion: Problems with the Act

The MCA 2005 criteria for assessing a person's decision-making capacity have been covered in the first part of this chapter. At first, these criteria seem to be quite clear, but there are some problems with the practical implementation of the test. First, there is an inherent danger in assuming that the test is straightforward. This might lead healthcare professionals simply to add capacity assessments to their service user's 'to-do' lists and regard them as a 'tick-box' exercise. Assessments might fall to more junior healthcare professionals without a good understanding of the process, creating potential for overriding a service user's autonomy, or being open to negligence. Good training and supervision of healthcare professionals in the subtleties of capacity assessment is essential. Online learning packages exist, provided by the National Health Service (NHS), but they reduce the information to rather dry detail. Face-to-face training or use of case scenarios allows for better discussion and exploration of the nuances of capacity assessment.

The second problem is the impact of time on the assessment process. Assessment of a person's ability to make a complex decision may take an hour or more, once a full discussion has been had. The assessor needs time to formulate an opinion and to document it. This can be difficult to achieve within the context of reduced staffing levels.

The third problem is related to the reduction of continuity in modern healthcare practice. We may be required to care for service users that are new to us and this poses an inherent problem when it comes to assessing their capacity. We need to know our service users well so that the capacity test is fair. We need to get to know them, their hopes, their views, and their desires in terms of treatment. It goes without saying that this takes time and that someone else might be better placed to undertake the assessment.

The fourth problem is about information and is related to the first, ensuring adequate training. We need to make sure that we have provided the fullest information, pitched at the appropriate level for the person, in order to assess their ability to make a decision. Too often we might give scant information and expect a person to make a life-changing choice. We need to prepare for the assessment and ensure that we know what information we are going to give before we do it.

The final problem relates to the physical environment in most acute hospitals. All too often there is no quiet space available to have these long and detailed discussions. On many occasions, service users have limited mobility and discussions have to be conducted at the bedside. This in itself can limit the quality of the assessment carried out.

So how does the legislation work in other areas of the UK?

Mental Capacity Act (Northern Ireland) 2016

The Mental Capacity Act (Northern Ireland) (MCA (NI)) was passed in May 2016 (Northern Ireland introduces mental capacity legislation, 2016) and has not yet come into force. At face value it appears to be very similar to the English and Welsh legislation but there are differences. It introduces a number of changes in relation to capacity assessment that are discussed in more detail below.

Removal of separate legislation covering decisions about mental health treatment

The Mental Health Order 1986 (NI) was a piece of legislation similar to the Mental Health Act. It made compulsory detention and treatment of people with mental disorder possible, regardless of their capacity to consent to this. The MCA (NI) removes this piece of legislation for people over 16 years of age, meaning that it will not be possible to compel people to detention and treatment if they have capacity to make a decision about it and refuse. Instead, such admission and treatment will be based upon the same 'best interests' process as for all other decisions in people that lack capacity (Ruck Keene, 2014). This is vastly different to English and Welsh law, where there is separate legislation, and is a significant change in the way in which people with mental health problems are treated and cared for.

A requirement to provide all practicable help and support

The Act sets out a number of principles that encompass capacity and best interests. The capacity principles in section 1(4) set out a requirement that a person cannot be held to lack capacity to make a decision, "...unless all practicable help and support ... have been given without success" (MCA NI 2016). This is a far more robust requirement, placed on the assessor, to assist people to make decisions (Ruck Keene, 2014). It goes on, in section 5, to stipulate what this level of support should be, with the caveat that they should be taken, "...so far as practicable" (MCA NI 2016):

> - Provision of, or explanation of, information relevant to the decision in a way appropriate to the person's circumstances. This must include information about the consequences of choosing different options and of making no decision at all. Information appropriate to circumstances might include:
>
> • Simple language, or visual aids
>
> • Support for communicating information or explanation.
>
> - Ensuring that the timing of the capacity assessment is at a time likely to help the person make it.
>
> - Ensuring that the capacity assessment is conducted in an environment that is likely to help the person make the decision.
>
> - Ensuring that help and support is given by people who are likely to help the person make a decision, in particular people who provide support to help the person communicate their decision.

These requirements not only set out a detailed explanation of what kind of support is needed, but also ask the assessor to try them and to demonstrate that they were not successful in assisting the person to make a decision. The England and Wales MCA (2005) requirements appear vague in comparison to these.

A change in the diagnostic threshold

The Act makes some subtle changes to the diagnostic threshold requirement. Section 3(1) still holds that a person must be unable to make a decision because of an impairment, or a disturbance in the functioning of, the mind or brain, but it widens the caveats linked to capacity assessment. There are the same safeguards about being unable to determine lack of capacity on the basis of any condition a person might have, but section 1(3)(b) widens the scope of other limits from age, appearance, or aspect of behaviour to "…any other characteristic of the person".

Section 3(2)(b) states that the cause of the disturbance is irrelevant and section 3(3) clarifies that it doesn't matter whether it is caused by a disorder, or disability, or otherwise.

A change in the functional test

The functional test is largely unchanged from the MCA 2005. There is an important difference, however, in the wording of two parts of the test. First, the requirement to retain information is expanded, at section 1(4)(b), to explain that it must be "…for the time required to make the decision" (MCA NI, 2016), whereas the MCA 2005, at section 3(1)(2) states that it should only be for a short period. Secondly, there is a change to the 'use and weigh' part of the test (MCA NI, 2016, 2016, s.4(1)):

> "…a person is "unable to make a decision … if [they]
>
> (c) [Are] not able to appreciate the relevance of that information and to use and weigh that information as part of the process of making the decision …"

The test expands to include the standard of appreciation, as discussed earlier in the chapter. Assessors have to consider whether the person's impairment affects their insight into the ability to carry out the decision. It provides more help in situations where the issue may not be related to frank cognitive difficulties, but related to subtle executive function, e.g., in Acquired Brain Injury (Ruck Keene, 2014). This also removes insight as an assumption of the function of understanding.

The Adults with Incapacity Act (Scotland) 2000

This Act received Royal Assent in May 2000 (Adults with Incapacity (Scotland) Act 2000) and contains some marked differences from the other pieces of UK legislation. As with the other Acts it applies to people aged 16 and over and sets out a presumption of capacity in making "personal decisions and managing their own affairs" (Adults with Incapacity (Scotland) Act 2000: Code of Practice (Third Edition), 2010, p. 3). It also holds that capacity is not an all-or-nothing matter but is decision-specific (Adults with Incapacity (Scotland) Act 2000: Code of Practice (Third Edition), 2010, p. 4). The Act covers incapacity in all settings, with a specific section covering health-related decisions. The following discussion focuses on this section. The capacity test is broadly similar in approach although any differences are discussed later, but first a look at the general principles of the Act as relevant to the capacity test.

General principles: Benefit and acquisition of new skills

The first general principle is one of benefit, holding that it is only possible to act on a person's behalf if an intervention is of benefit to them (Adults with Incapacity (Scotland) Act 2000, 2000, s.1(2)). This principle does not seem to apply to the capacity assessment itself, but the Code of Practice extends it to include deferring the decision if reasonably possible, until the person regains sufficient capacity to make it (Adults with Incapacity (Scotland) Act 2000: Code of Practice (Third Edition), 2010, p. 4).

The Act also sets out a requirement to encourage the person to exercise whatever skills he or she might have and to try to develop new skills in doing this (Adults with Incapacity (Scotland) Act 2000, 2000, s.1(5)). This is different to the other legislation, which aims to involve the person but not to enable them to acquire new decision-making powers.

Medical decisions

Section 47 of the Act covers decisions related to medical treatment and research. It applies when a medial practitioner primarily responsible for the person's medical treatment decides that they are 'incapable' in relation to making a decision about a particular medical treatment (Adults with Incapacity (Scotland) Act 2000, s.47(1)). Section 47(3) explains that they can delegate their authority to any other person, i.e., allied health professionals, so long as they act on their behalf or with their approval. Medical treatment has a wide definition and is held to be "…any procedure or treatment designed to safeguard or promote physical or mental health" (Adults with Incapacity (Scotland) Act 2000, s.47(4)). If the person lacks capacity then the medical practitioner, or their delegate, has authority to do "…what is reasonable in the circumstances, in relation to the medical treatment, to safeguard or promote the physical or mental health of the adult" (Adults with Incapacity (Scotland) Act 2000, s.47(2)). They must still ensure that they encourage the person to make decisions about other aspects of their care (Adults with Incapacity (Scotland) Act 2000: Code of Practice (Third Edition), 2010). They cannot place the person in hospital for treatment of mental disorder against their will using this test as it falls under separate mental health legislation.

The medical practitioner must still assess capacity. The test is similar to those in the other Acts, as it has both a diagnostic and a functional test. The elements of these are worth considering in more detail.

The functional test

The functional test, in section 1(6), holds that for someone to lack capacity (in the words of the Act be "incapable" (Adults with Incapacity (Scotland) Act 2000, 2000)), they must be unable to:

- Act; or

- Make decisions; or

- Communicate decisions; or

- Understand decisions; or

- Retain the memory of decisions.

The implication is that an inability to undertake any one part, in relation to a decision, means that a person lacks capacity to make that decision. The inclusion of the test of being able to act is different to the other two statutes and perhaps satisfies the problem of capacity assessment in people with dys-executive function, also covered by NI law but in a different way. If people are able of making a decision but are unable to carry it out, then they might still be held to be lacking capacity.

The Code of Practice (2010) expands on the requirements of understanding, similar to the other Acts, and based on the BMA's 2003 guidance on capacity and consent. There are, however, a couple of key differences in that:

- The person has to be given "every possible assistance" to understand their own medical condition and the decision that is required (Adults with Incapacity (Scotland) Act 2000: Code of Practice (Third Edition), para 1.11). This is different to all practicable assistance.

- The person has to know that the information is of personal relevance to them.

- They must know that they have the right to refuse and know how to do this.

- The assessor must check whether the person has expressed any relevant wishes in the past.

- The assessor must check that the view expressed now is consistent with "…their previously preferred moral, cultural, family, and experiential background".

- The assessor must check that there is no coercion (Adults with Incapacity (Scotland) Act 2000: Code of Practice (Third Edition), para 1.22).

It also sets out a clear standard against which to measure capacity. The person should not be held to any societal norm of decision making, but should be compared to what is normal for them. This means the assessor should draw on their own knowledge of the person and that of relatives and other professionals, in order to determine whether there has been a change in their capacity (Adults with Incapacity (Scotland) Act 2000: Code of Practice (Third Edition), para 1.16).

The assessor has to consider the complexity of the decision in the assessment and also look at barriers to autonomous decision making, including (Adults with Incapacity (Scotland) Act 2000: Code of Practice (Third Edition), para 1.24):

- sensory/physical impairment

- suggestibility

- the effects of alcohol, drugs, or medication

- fatigue

- pain

- mental health status.

Finally, there is a requirement to involve clinical psychologists and SLTs where the incapacity relates to communication skills. This is part of the "absolute obligation to facilitating the exercise of capacity, where possible" (Adults with Incapacity (Scotland) Act 2000: Code of Practice (Third Edition), para 1.25).

The diagnostic test

The diagnostic test is satisfied if the person is unable to meet the functional test due to a 'mental disorder' or due to a physical disability causing inability to communicate (Adults with Incapacity (Scotland) Act 2000, s.1(6)). The definition of 'mental disorder' comes from the Mental Health Care and Treatment (Scotland) Act 2003 (Adults with Incapacity (Scotland) Act 2000: Code of Practice (Third Edition), para 1.21). Section 328(1) defines this as "...any mental illness, personality disorder, or learning disability, however caused or manifested". There is a caveat within this section, designed to avoid discriminating against people with communication difficulties. It says that a person does not satisfy the test if their communication impairment can be made good by the aid of a person or a machine. The aid can be of an interpretative nature or otherwise (Adults with Incapacity (Scotland) Act 2000, s.1(6)).

The Code of Practice (2010, para 1.21) clarifies that this is not a threshold met by a particular diagnosis, lifestyle, behaviour, or status. It even allows for unwise decision making, as in the other Acts. It holds that the person cannot be considered mentally disordered on grounds of:

- sexual orientation or sexual deviancy

- transsexualism or transvestitism

- alcohol or drug dependence

- behaviour that either causes or is likely to cause harassment, alarm, or distress to any others

- acting as no prudent person would act.

Finally the Code of Practice (2010, para 1.9) gives a prescriptive list of things that do not denote incapacity (see Table 1.1), explaining that it is not possible to assume incapacity on the basis of a person's diagnosis, behaviour, or situation, even if they have a mental disorder. In this way, it encourages an assessment of capacity that is fair and based on the ability to make a decision.

Conclusion

This chapter has described and compared the three pieces of legislation that cover assessment of capacity in the UK. These all incorporate a similar

Table 1.1 Situations that do not denote a lack of capacity.

Being in community care	Promiscuity
Psychotic illness	Brain injury
Dementia, especially early stage	Physical disability
Speech or writing problems	Criminal convictions/offence
Addiction	Acquired or progressive neurological condition
Disagreeing with treatment or people	Declining advice
proposing it	Rejecting a recommendation on emotional
Learning disability	rather than rational grounds
Adult at risk	
Irrational behaviour	

approach: being decision-specific, setting out a functional test, and a diagnostic threshold. There are subtle differences in the functional tests that might yield different outcomes for a person depending on where they are tested. In spite of detail provided in codes of practice there is potential for subjective variation in outcome, based on the assessor and their reading of the tests. The process described is neither simple, nor is it perfect. It is ever-changing, guided by new insights provided by case law.

In addition to this there is a movement towards reform. The United Nations Convention on the Rights of Persons with Disabilities (CRPD) is a treaty that the UK has signed, ratified, and is legally bound to. It is a framework designed to achieve universal rights protection for people with disabilities. One of the rights is the right to legal capacity on an equal basis (UNCRPD Article 12 - Equal recognitions before the law, 2006), meaning the right to be a legal agent whose decisions are respected and validated by law. Although the CRPD does not mention the issue of mental capacity, it can be a basis for granting legal capacity for certain decisions (Series, Arstein-Kerslake, Gooding, & Flynn, pp. 2, 5). The three UK statues all contain a diagnostic threshold based on some form of impairment. The CRPD questions a system that might deny legal capacity based on this approach. The England and Wales MCA 2005 has come under particular scrutiny as its 'functional test approach' can be applied in a discriminatory way to people with disabilities, as people with disabilities are more likely to have the test applied to them than those that do not (Series et al., p.6). In addition, there are concerns that the provision of support in the Act is to help a person pass the test, whereas the Committee hold that support should be available, "regardless of 'mental capacity'" (UNCRPD Article 12 - Equal recognitions before the law, 2006, para 25(i)). The CRPD holds that we should avoid testing capacity, with the resultant substituted decision-making if a person is unable to make a decision. It suggests that a person is supported and encouraged to make their decisions for themselves (Richardson, 2013, p. 92). Whilst Scottish and Northern Irish legislation makes some moves towards this standard, English and Welsh law may well not meet it. The issues raised by the CRPD, combined with the House of Lords' post-legislative scrutiny (Select Committee on the Mental Capacity Act 2005, Report of Session 2013-14), and the impact of case law, means that mental capacity law is likely to experience reform in the future.

References

Adults with Incapacity (Scotland) Act 2000. (2000, May 9). Retrieved from: legislation.gov. uk: http://www.legislation.gov.uk/asp/2000/4/introduction

Adults with Incapacity (Scotland) Act 2000: Code of Practice (Third Edition). (2010, October 20). Retrieved from Scottish Government: http://www.gov.scot/ Publications/2010/10/20153801/0

Applebaum, P.S. & Grisso, T. (1995, April). The MacArthur Treatment Competence Study. I. *Law and Human Behaviour, 19*(2), 105-126. doi:10.1007/BF01499321

Brazier, M. & Cave, E. (2007). *Medicine, Patients and the Law, 4th Edition.* London: Penguin.

CRPD, U. N. (2014, April 11). *General Comment No.1 - Article 12: Equal recognition before the law.* Retrieved August 01, 2017, from United Nations: https://documents-dds-ny. un.org/doc/UNDOC/GEN/G14/031/20/PDF/G1403120.pdf?OpenElement

Department for Constitutional Affairs. (2007). *Mental Capacity Act 2005 Code of Practice.* London: The Stationery Office.

Grisso, T. & Applebaum, P.S. (1998). *Assessing Competence to Consent to Treatment.* Oxford: Oxford University Press.

Heart of England NHS Foundation Trust vs JB, [2014] EWCOP 342 (COP) (2014) 137 BMLR 232 (Court of Protection February 17, 2014). doi:http://www.bailii.org/ew/cases/ EWHC/COP/2014/342.html

Hope, T. (2004). *Medical Ethics: A Very Short Introduction.* Oxford: Oxford University Press.

House of Lords. (2014). *Select Committee on the Mental Capacity Act 2005, Report of Session 2013-14.* London: Authority of the House of Lords. Retrieved from https://publications. parliament.uk/pa/ld201314/ldselect/ldmentalcap/139/139.pdf

Jackson, E. (2006). *Medical Law Text, Cases, and Materials.* Oxford: Oxford University Press.

Kings College Hospital NHS Foundation Trust and C and V, [2015] EWCOP 80 (2016) COPLR 50 (Court of Protection November 30, 2015). Retrieved August 01, 2017, from http://www.bailii.org/ew/cases/EWCOP/2015/80.html

Mental Capacity Act (Northern Ireland) 2016. (2016, May 9). Retrieved from legislation. gov.uk: http://www.legislation.gov.uk/nia/2016/18/contents

Mental Capacity Act 2005. (n.d.). Retrieved August 01, 2017, from Legislation.gov.uk: http:// www.legislation.gov.uk/ukpga/2005/9/contents

Northern Ireland introduces mental capacity legislation. (2016, August 23). Retrieved August 01, 2017, from Headway: https://www.headway.org.uk/news/national-news/northern-ireland-introduces-mental-capacity-legislation/

Raymont, V., Bingley, W., Buchanan, A., David, A.D., Hayward, P., Wessely, S., & Hotopf, M. (2004, October 16-22). Prevalence of mental incapacity in medical inpatients and associated risk factors: cross sectional study. *The Lancet, 364*(9443), 1421-1427. doi:10.1016/S0410-6736(04)17224-3

Richardson, G. (2013). Mental capacity in the shadow of suicide: What can the law do? *International Journal of Law in Context, 9*(1), 87. doi:10.1017/S174455231200050X

Ruck Keene, A. (2014, July 3). *Throwing down the gauntlet - the mental capacity revolution in Northern Ireland.* Retrieved from Mental Capacity Law and Policy: http://www.mentalcapacitylawandpolicy.org.uk/throwing-down-the-gauntlet-the-mental-capacity-revolution-in-northern-ireland/

Ruck Keene, A. (2017). Is mental capacity in the eye of the beholder? *Advances in Mental Health and Intellectual Disabilities, 11*(2), 30-39. doi:10.1108/AMHID-11-2016-0035

Ruck Keene, A., Butler-Cole, V., Allen, N., Bicarregui, A., Kohn, N., & Akhtar, S. (2016, August 1). *A Brief Guide to Carrying Out Capacity Assessments.* Retrieved August 01, 2017, from Mental Capacity Law and Policy: http://www.39essex.com/content/wp-content/uploads/2016/08/Capacity-Assessments-Guide-August-2016.pdf

Series, L., Arstein-Kerslake, A., Gooding, P., & Flynn, E. (n.d.). Retrieved from ThirtyNine Essex Street: http://www.39essex.com/docs/newsletters/crpd_discussion_paper_series_et_al.pdf

UNCRPD Article 12 - Equal recognitions before the law. (2006, December 13). Retrieved August 01, 2017, from United Nations Division for Social Policy and Development Disability: https://www.un.org/development/desa/disabilities/convention-on-the-rights-of-persons-with-disabilities/article-12-equal-recognition-before-the-law.html

2 Training speech and language therapists

Anna Volkmer and Isla Jones

Introduction

The delivery of all modern healthcare, including speech and language therapy, is founded on evidence-based practice. However, given the busy clinical environment, it can be extremely challenging for professionals to keep up-to-date with the current evidence base. The Mental Capacity Act (MCA, 2005) may pose additional barriers for healthcare clinicians such as speech and language therapists (SLTs). It is written in a litigious style that may feel intimidating and complex. It may even feel as though it ought not fall into a SLT's clinical role to be reading this material.

Nevertheless, SLTs are increasingly encountering clinical issues related to decision-making mental capacity. They are becoming involved in assessments of decision making; for example, supporting a person's communication (particularly comprehension) during assessment by someone else; or else directly assessing the decision-making capacity of individuals (particularly where it relates to their swallow function). SLTs are also seeing growing numbers of service users with progressive communication difficulties such as dementia, MS, MND, Parkinson's disease and so forth. In therapy sessions SLTs are increasingly discussing plans for future decision making. As the diseases progress and individuals are no longer able to make decisions, SLTs are also being involved in best interests' decisions.

In Section 1 of this chapter this new and evolving role for SLTs is discussed in more detail. Different training methods are considered in relation to supporting SLTs to improve their knowledge and understanding within their teams (both departmental and more broadly). Case studies and vignettes are provided in Section 2, alongside reflective tools to enable the planning and delivery of training sessions on this topic.

Section I: Why should SLTs be involved in decision making and the Mental Capacity Act (2005)?

"...a person lacks capacity in relation to a matter if at the material time he is unable to make a decision for himself in relation to the matter because of an impairment of, or a disturbance in the functioning of, the mind or the brain." (MCA 2005, Section 2, 1)

The MCA (2005) was written to protect vulnerable adults ("those with an impairment of, or a disturbance in the functioning of, the mind or brain") including those living with the consequences of a stroke or brain injury, who have dementia, schizophrenia, delirium, concussion, or are suffering the consequence of drugs or alcohol use. These are also typically clients who may be seen by an SLT in the clinical setting. SLTs provide assessment, management and intervention for adults with communication difficulties. These communication difficulties may be the result of a stroke, brain injury, progressive neurological conditions such as Parkinson's disease, multiple sclerosis or motor neurone disease. There are also many SLTs employed in adult mental health services working with people with dementia, schizophrenia and many other mental health conditions.

All the conditions described above can result in difficulties that may affect an individual's ability to make decisions. This may include their ability to understand the relevant information, retain this information, weigh up said information and, finally, their ability to communicate their decision. As described in Chapter 1, these are the four key domains of the functional test of decision-making ability in the MCA (2005).

In its recent response to the draft Mental Capacity Bill for Northern Ireland, The Royal College of Speech and Language Therapy (RCSLT) emphasised that speech, language and communication skills are essential for maintaining relationships, understanding social contexts, expressing individuality and exercising choice and control over personal decisions (RCSLT, 2014). The RCSLT is clear in emphasising that SLTs have a key role in the assessment of decision-making capacity. The recent RCSLT factsheet on mental capacity states that SLTs "...promote inclusion, dignity, choice, and equality of access to services. They also reduce the potential risk of people with communication needs being wrongly deemed as lacking capacity and, in some extreme cases, being deprived of their liberty..." (RCSLT, 2017 Factsheet, p. 1).

Internationally, many speech and language researchers have advocated that SLTs (Speech and Language Pathologists; SLPs) be involved in capacity assessments. Canadian authors Suleman and Hopper (2016) emphasise that "It is an ethical imperative that healthcare professionals determine the best ways to assess decision-making capacity so that an individual's right to autonomy and self-determination is not unnecessarily revoked. [...] SLPs have a specialised professional skill set that can help individuals with aphasia reveal their true decision-making capacity. As such, to accurately determine whether an individual with aphasia is able to make autonomous choice, it is crucial that SLPs be involved in the team assessment of decision-making capacity" (Suleman & Hopper, 2016, p.394). In the UK McCormick et al (2017) recommend that "training SLTs on decision-making and capacity assessment should be an integral part of curriculum in SLT programmes" (McCormick, Bose, & Marinis, 2017). In Australia, Zuscak, Peisah, and Ferguson (2015) describe specific specialist communication tools and skills an SLT can use to ensure all practicable steps have been used to support individuals with aphasia in decision making.

Many people with communication difficulties can demonstrate capacity to make decisions with the correct 'practicable steps', i.e., communication supports. With the right communication support they are able to exercise their right to choose and make their own decisions (RCSLT, 2014a). The MCA 2005 Code of Practice (2007) and the General Medical Council (2013) recommend seeking the professional opinion of an SLT to support capacity assessments of individuals with communication difficulties. In fact, SLTs are identified within the Adults with Incapacity Codes of Practice in Scotland (2010) as specialists in assessing and advising on capacity to understand and communicate informed decisions.

The RCSLT also advocates strongly for SLTs to be involved in assessments of decision-making capacity for people with communication difficulties. They have outlined some of the suggested specifics of this role in documents such as the "Submission from the Royal College of Speech and Language Therapists to the Department of Health, Social Services and Public Safety and the Department of Justice's Consultation on proposals for the Draft Mental Capacity Bill, Northern Ireland (2014a)", "RCSLT Mental Health Strategy for Scotland 2011–2015: A consultation". The RCSLT has also issued a number of position papers on Speech and Language Therapy in Critical Care (2014b) and Speech and Language Therapy for People with

Dementia (2014c), which provide specific commentary on the SLT's role in these conditions.

In Canada and Australia, the speech and language therapy practice associations have published professional guidelines outlining the different roles of the SLT in mental capacity assessments. At the time of writing, the RCSLT is currently in the process of developing its web pages and writing a specific position statement on the role of the SLT in decision making and mental capacity. Not only will this formalise the role of SLTs, but it will provide much-needed confidence, empowerment and guidance to current practitioners.

Barriers to SLTs being involved in capacity assessments

Many healthcare services recognise that there are barriers to providing SLT services when there is an issue related to mental capacity. The issues may be as simple as a lack of resources, or as complex and seemingly insurmountable as a lack of awareness of the SLT role in the wider health community. Yet many barriers are within the discipline itself. SLTs are often concerned about being involved in assessments of decision-making capacity. This may be for a variety of reasons, including a lack of confidence in carrying out the assessment, concerns about the conflict in role, or a lack of time and resources (Volkmer, 2016). McCormick et al. (2017) surveyed 56 SLTs across England working with people with aphasia around their knowledge and awareness of the MCA, their involvement with capacity assessments and their training needs. The results of this survey are extremely pertinent to this discussion. Survey respondents reported a lack of knowledge of the MCA, a lack of resources to conduct assessments and a lack of confidence in carrying out these assessments (McCormick et al., 2017). The authors also report qualitative responses from SLTs, which identify concerns regarding a lack of basic MCA training within their trusts, difficulties in managing conflict and requiring training in this area, as well as a broader lack of understanding and respect for the assistance the SLT can offer to other professionals. Another significant concern for respondents was the lack of evidence-based resources for SLTs to use in supporting their involvement in capacity assessments. Although most respondents reported being involved in a limited number of capacity assessments, very few had regular involvement.

McCormick et al. (2017) emphasise the likelihood that SLTs are routinely underutilised in capacity assessments due to a lack of awareness of the SLT role amongst other professions. This echoes literature published in Canada (Carling-Rowland et al., 2010) and Australia (Aldous et al., 2014) where the capacity act legislation and the role of the SLT are considered comparable to England and Wales. This finding is not surprising given the broader lack of awareness of the SLT role in communication. A recent UK-wide survey found that a significant barrier for people with language-led dementias accessing SLT services was the lack of awareness of the SLT role amongst the wider health community (Volkmer, Spector, Warren et al., 2018).

Aldous et al. (2014) surveyed 59 SLTs working with adults with aphasia in Australia on current practices, satisfaction and confidence in participating in capacity assessments. SLT respondents reported feeling undervalued and dissatisfied with current assessment procedures for capacity. SLTs in Australia found the process difficult and time-consuming and did not feel that their professional training had adequately prepared them for their role. Suleman and Hopper (2016) interviewed 16 SLTs working with aphasia in Alberta, Canada, who reported similar barriers to delivering services. The qualitative analysis of the interviews revealed that SLTs felt other professionals didn't understand the breadth of their role and had a "very narrow view of what we do". They also highlighted concerns regarding their large workloads and raised the issue of how the profession represents itself.

In all these studies, SLTs report a need for training (Aldous et al., 2014; McCormick et al., 2017; Suleman & Hopper, 2016). This includes both discipline-specific and multidisciplinary training. McCormick et al. (2017) emphasise that "improving the outcome of capacity assessment for PWA [people with aphasia] would require education and information regarding the impact of language difficulties on decision-making and capacity assessments for care professionals as well as for SLTs" (McCormick et al., 2017, p. 11). Training can in turn raise the awareness of the role of the SLT amongst other professionals. It is worth commenting that these studies were all focused on SLTs working with aphasia; there is even less known of the current practices in the wider profession. Yet capacity assessment is an issue arising across all adult and frequently some paediatric SLT caseloads. Thus, it presents as a core clinical competence and many SLTs would likely benefit from specific training in this area of practice.

The role of the SLT in assessments of decision making

It is irrefutable that SLTs should be involved in the decision-making process in some way. Ferguson, Duffield, and Worrall (2010) and Suleman and Hopper (2016) have interviewed SLTs in Australia and Canada and their research has highlighted the breadth and variety of the SLT role in decision-making assessments. They describe how SLTs 'can act as "assessors" (i.e., assess an individual's language and communication), "advocates" (i.e., assert the individual's rights and autonomy), "consultants" (i.e., provide professional assessments of an individual's decision-making abilities), "interpreters" or "translators" (i.e., facilitate the delivery of messages from the individual being assessed), "educators" (i.e., teach information), "facilitators" (i.e., indirectly assist or guide), "therapists" (i.e., provide speech, language, or communication intervention), "mediators" (i.e., assist in conflict resolution), "leaders" (i.e., manage other people), and "negotiators" (i.e., facilitate compromise)' (Suleman & Hopper, 2016, p. 383).

The members of the Southern Psychiatry of Old Age Clinical Excellence Network (CEN) agree that SLTs should be involved in mental capacity assessments in England and that they play a variety of roles in the process. Their descriptions of some of these roles are listed in Table 2.1.

The RCSLT has expanded on this and highlighted what it believes to be the clear role of the SLT. This includes to:

- "undertake in-depth, detailed assessments of an individual's current, and likely future, ability to communicate, including their ability to understand, express themselves, retain and recall information, and reason (weigh up different options)

- carry out capacity assessments themselves and/or contribute to multidisciplinary capacity assessments of people with communication needs

- support people with communication needs to demonstrate their decision-making capacity

- support people who cannot make informed decisions to express their preferences and wishes in relation to any decision made on their behalf

Table 2.1 Role of SLTs in capacity assessments described by described by Southern Psychiatry of Old Age Clinical Excellence Network (Devereux et al., 2016).

SLTs as assessors As an assessor, an SLT may work with a client over a number of sessions in order to assess their decision-making abilities in relation to understanding, retention, weighing up the issue and expressing themselves. This assessment may often be conducted alongside other professionals. Assessment will likely include an assessment of the individual's preferences, regardless of whether they are deemed to lack capacity. Assessing capacity can include checking on previous advance care plans and any power of attorney that may have been donated. The assessor must understand the decision in question and the options. Meeting the client informally and conducting formal assessments to establish communication needs and supports prior to the formal capacity assessment can be useful. This can ensure that the SLT uses the appropriate measures during the assessment to support the client. On completing the assessment, the SLT should document the outcome, together the measures used and the evidence for the outcome for the assessment. This should be clearly communicated to both the team and the client being assessed.
SLTs as decision makers As a decision maker, the SLT is the person who takes action if the client does not have capacity. This will be relevant to decisions around diet modification (risk feeding) and augmentative and alternative communication choices. These sessions will require the SLT to provide relevant information in an accessible way to ensure the client is able to engage in expressing their preferences even if they lack capacity. As with the role of assessor, the SLT needs to demonstrate having sought evidence, provided appropriate information, clear documentation and communication throughout. An SLT may act as an assessor on issues other than those described, alongside another clinician even when they are not the decision maker.
SLTs as advocates An SLT may act as an advocate for existing clients with whom the SLT already has a relationship in order to help them express their views or provide evidence of their views and wishes. This may involve explaining communication difficulties or needs to the assessor and decision maker in order to optimize the assessment process. Advocating may also involve communicating preferences someone has communicated at another time, for example during a therapy session. We may be most likely to act as an advocate in a best interest decision meeting.
SLTs as educators or trainers An educator or trainer may act to support clients in preparing them for the assessment and decision to be made or may act to support other professionals through training or provision of aids to enable communication during an assessment. This role may overlap with the role of a facilitator, where an SLT directly supports the client being assessed by, for example, accessing information in order to make a choice or in communicating a decision or preference.
Multiplicity of roles As a CEN, we acknowledge that SLTs may take on different roles within the mental capacity assessment process at different times. We may therefore need to take on several of the above roles with any one client during the course of their care. We are of the opinion that assessments may be done with another professional from our or another discipline, or with family members present.

- advise and train people on the best means by which someone with a communication disability might overcome their disability so they can make and communicate informed decisions about their treatment and care

- support people to understand how to communicate with individuals who have been found to lack decision-making capacity" (RCSLT, 2017, Mental Capacity Factsheet).

Concerns have been raised around the risk in taking on these roles and the impact this can have, such as jeopardising a therapeutic relationship with the client that may be essential to their rehabilitation (Volkmer, 2016). These considerations are valid; however, as with any clinical endeavour or activity, they should be prioritised and evaluated in terms of broader clinical risk. There may be some situations where another team member is equally or better placed to take on a role that could impact negatively on a therapeutic relationship. Equally, should there be no other appropriate professional, it may be that the assessment of capacity is the priority for this individual; going home may be more important than their naming exercises. This sounds rather flippant, but needs to be carefully considered in practice.

Zuscak et al. (2016) go into further detail in their article and summarise the specific skills that an SLT can bring to a capacity assessment. They outline each of the four areas commonly considered key for decision making in legislation and discuss communication skills, aids and methods to enable people with aphasia to engage in this process. It is a useful article to refer to as an SLT but may also be useful for other professionals who are not convinced by the SLT role. A neat summary table from the article provides an overview of this (Table 2.2).

Upskilling a speech and language therapy department

The bulk of this book provides a resource on the role of the SLT in terms of training others in communication skills to support decision making and mental capacity. Chapter 3 provides a detailed description of training around capacity assessments in a healthcare setting. However, SLTs working

Table 2.2 Suggested alternative and augmentative communication methods for receptive and expressive language deficits (from Zuscak et al., 2016, p.1108).

Communication deficit	Capacity consideration	Communication strategies
Receptive language	(i) Understand the relevant information.	Repeat information in different ways. Check for comprehension. Seek advice from SLP regarding nature of difficulties (i.e., rise time and noise build-up) and deficit-specific strategies.
Expressive language General cognitive impairment	(iv) Communicate a choice.	Use fixed choice response options. Verify responses through repetition, expansion and summarising. Attend to nonverbal cues for signs of intended meaning. Use the favoured mode of communication. Use attentive and active listening. Seek advice from SLP regarding: - Use of communication boards, gesture, pantomime, drawing and pointing. - Possible alternatives such as speech synthesisers. - SLP support for communication partner before and/or during interaction.
	(ii) Appreciate the nature, significance and likely consequences of the decision being made.	Keep language simple. Allow plenty of time. Use all available aids. Revisit important decisions over time. Liaise with families. Seek SLP advice for:
	(iii) Reason about the choices.	- Strategies for assessment team to support decision-making. - Assessment with non-linguistic cognitive tests.

with adults must prioritise an understanding of not only decision-making capacity but also advance planning and best interests' decision-making. These are interlinked areas that influence one another, and clinicians require an insight as to how this affects their clinical practice. To assess the level of knowledge within your department it may be best to start by investigating this before launching into anything further. Table 2.3 provides an example of a checklist to ascertain the training needs within the team and plan the most appropriate and relevant training.

It is also vitally important to consider the pastoral and emotional needs of staff members and SLTs in relation to this topic. Capacity is an area that staff may simply wish to debrief on. They may be searching for

Table 2.3 Checklist to ascertain the training needs within the team.

Example questions you might include in a brief pretraining questionnaire or feedback form	Area of focus for your training
Have you done the mandatory organizational Mental Capacity Training? Who is the mental capacity lead in the service/ trust? Where do you find information on mental capacity? What is safeguarding?	Level 1: Basic information and interpretation of what the mental capacity is and your local guidance (mandatory training should cover this).
What is an advanced plan? Have you been involved in a capacity assessment? If yes to the above question – how many assessments have you been involved in? Who (else) is involved in assessments of decision making and mental capacity where you work? Is there a specific process or *procedure* for carrying out a mental capacity assessment where you work? What do you do if you don't agree with the outcome of a mental capacity assessment carried out by a colleague? What role(s) might you take when one of your clients requires a mental capacity assessment? What does best interest decision making mean?	Level 2: Extended training considering the individual's and the team's role and how this may affect various clinical situations. Lots of case examples may be useful. Much of this could be covered in multidisciplinary team training to maximise the impact around role and communication styles.
What is the difference between the MCA (2005) and the Mental Health Act? What is Deprivation of Liberty? What do you have to do with the Court of Protection?	Level 3: More complex training requiring in-depth and up-to-date discussion on current legislation and case law (will likely need an expert in current legislation to deliver this, e.g., your capacity lead).
SLT specific What tools do you use when assessing people in relation to their mental capacity? What tools or resources do you use to support people in mental capacity assessments? What tools or resources do you use to support people in relation to advance planning, etc? How do you prioritise an issue related to capacity on an SLT caseload?	Level 3: Discipline-specific training to discuss and pool resources and ideas, agree strategies and local service structures.
What do you hope to address in the session? Do you have any specific concerns regarding decision making and mental capacity? Would you like to provide example case studies or scenarios that you would be interested and willing to discuss?	Level 3: More in-depth exploration of cases may be best managed in smaller groups, perhaps within regular peer supervision groups or regular smaller team meetings. These issues may equally be addressed within the broader discipline, e.g., at a specific CEN, for example.

a forum for case discussion and problem solving, or an opportunity to ensure they are 'following the rules'. As previously emphasised, capacity can be an intimidating area of practice and staff may wish to share stories and frustrations. Individuals may even find that they wish to discuss issues affecting them in their own lives (their own family or friends) or issues may conflict with their personal values and beliefs. It can be difficult to see a service user's will and preferences as 'the right decision' if they are directly opposing your own beliefs. Being open and honest about all these concerns, as per the recommendations in the MCA 2005 Code of Practice (2007), will improve communication within teams and thus improve service user care.

Planning your training

Resources

Health professionals need to understand their responsibilities in decision-making capacity in terms of the MCA. Not understanding this can result in (a) inconsistent practices within and between services and more seriously b) errors and omissions in service user care. The House of Commons (2014) report on implementation of the MCA reflected some of the issues; it found that healthcare staff were not familiar with the MCA and what this meant in terms of their service users. This report recommended the development of the national NICE SCIE guidelines on decision-making and mental capacity for health and social care professionals (forthcoming October 2018 at the time of writing). The NICE SCIE guidelines will be the most relevant resource to refer to alongside the MCA (2005) itself and the MCA Code of Practice (2007). Additionally, SCIE has a host of useful and relevant additional resources and online materials to complement this.

Every trust and organization will likely have its own policy on how it expects its employees to deal with mental capacity. National Health Service (NHS) employees are expected to undertake mandatory training on mental capacity that should cover issues such as consent (this has been the focus of recent legislative changes in 2017 and is particularly relevant). Many health services now also have mental capacity leads whose role is to liaise with, and support staff in their practice. There are many resources available and more currently in development to support health and social care professionals.

Table 2.4 Basic resources that SLTs can use for guidance: Have you looked at these documents?

Resources	Brief description	Do you have this document?
SLT-specific resources RCSLT position paper	Forthcoming: check the RCSLT website to ensure you are able to access this when available.	
RCSLT fact sheet	The RCSLT factsheet provides a useful and accessible overview of how an SLT may be involved in capacity assessment – accessible via the RCLST website.	
RCSLT website	The RCSLT website (member section) provides resources, guidance, advice and links to other relevant pages such as the inclusive communication pages.	
Local organizational resources Trust or organizational policy	Organizations may provide guidance on the expectations of their staff including information on documentation, conflict resolutions and information leaflets for service users.	
SLT Service Policy	SLT services may have developed their own guidelines to support prioritization of issues related to capacity.	
Generic resources MCA 2005	This is the most important document in relation to mental capacity and all health professionals must be aware of it and what it means.	
MCA 2005 Code of Practice 2007	The Code of Practice is a helpful document that interprets the MCA in a more accessible format. It provides case examples and specific suggestions on how the MCA can be implemented in the workplace. However, it doesn't provide much discipline-specific advice.	
NICE SCIE guidelines on decision making and mental capacity, 2018	The NICE SCIE guidelines will summarize the current evidence on capacity issues, providing recommendations using both the research and expert consultation. All health professionals should be aware of the document and use it to guide their practice.	

See Table 2.4 for a list of useful resources - you may wish to use this as a checklist to ensure you and your trainees are familiar with, and have access, to them. These are guidelines that professionals should be able to access to support their clinical practice. A simple start may be making these available in your department for independent professional development and to support clinical practice.

As previously mentioned, at the time of writing, the RCSLT is in the process of putting together a set of resources and a position paper. The RCSLT should be the first port of call for specific discipline advice and guidance. As our professional body, it can advocate for more consistent and equitable SLT services across the UK.

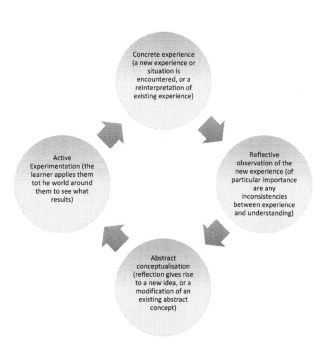

Figure 2.1 Kolb's model of learning (1984).

Learning styles

SLTs need to understand what the MCA (2005) means in terms of their daily clinical role and the service users they are working with. Professionals often have concerns about undertaking new tasks and may feel they are not proficient in a new area. As a result, some may avoid it, some may dive straight in, while others may research it thoroughly before they even try. These different learning styles are all valid. There have been studies examining how allied health students learn best, many of which are based around specific models of learning. Kolb's model of learning (1984) is a common framework applied in these studies. Kolb theorizes that there are four main stages to learning. He describes learning as a cycle whereby the individual experiences something, reflects on it and learns something that they then apply experimentally to the world around them (see Figure 2.1).

Individual's learning styles will vary depending on how they approach the situation, and what they think and how they feel about it. That said, they will still benefit from completing the entire learning cycle. Kolb proposes four different approaches to learning:

1. **Diverging** (feeling/watching): These are people who prefer to watch and gather information, before planning their approach.

2. **Assimilating** (watching/thinking): These are people who prefer to hear the theory, to listen to the explanation. They enjoy formal lectures and are analytical thinkers.

3. **Converging** (doing/thinking): These are people who like to solve problems and find solutions to practical issues.

4. **Accommodating** (doing/feeling): These are more likely to experiment, learning through concrete experience, and are the most 'hands-on'. They prefer to act on intuition than logic.

Hauer, Straub and Wolf (2004) found that SLT students in their cohort had a preference for an accommodating learning style (concrete experience to guide their learning). Other researchers have also found a preference for concrete experience amongst nursing students and mature students (Laschinger & Boss, 1984). This means they are able to use their feelings and experiences to change their behaviour in response to the situation. More recently, researchers have examined learning styles across different cultural groups in allied health students in Australia and Kuwait. These have revealed differing preferences for converging learning style in Australian students (Zoghi et al., 2010) and assimilating style in Arab cultures (Manee, Nadar, & Jahrami, 2013). It may be a useful exercise to understand the learning style of the individuals within your department. It is likely that not all SLTs will have the exact same approach to learning. What type of learner are you? What type of learners are there in your department? If you have a preference for concrete experiences then perhaps this is where the learning should start; by sharing what you have learned from your experiences. It can be useful to carry out a survey or hold a discussion on learning styles before you start. Perhaps begin simply by circulating the descriptions and asking people to identify how they feel they learn. Further, more in-depth and thorough evaluations of learning styles are available, including those written by Kolb himself, should these be of interest.

Alternatively, simply inviting staff to provide feedback on how they feel the team members could best develop their skills in this area is a good way of maximizing 'buy-in' and allowing everyone to feel that they are going to benefit from the session or training. This type of person-centred training is not significantly different to clinical practice.

Alternatively, it may be useful to form a scoping group or working party to decide and plan an extensive training or competency building exercise. Scoping groups meet to identify the breadth of a project and the questions that need answering or tasks that need to be undertaken. This approach can ensure learning is designed to meet everyone's needs.

Who will you deliver your training to?

The interdisciplinary team

Having graduated from university with a clinical and academic qualification, SLTs tend to be employed by and work within teams. Practitioners working with adults are also highly likely to be working not only in an SLT team, but in a multidisciplinary team (MDT). You will be assessing and managing people as a team. Frenk et al. (2010) highlight that this is a phase where teams of health professionals learn and deliver healthcare together, thus training needs to be tailored to the team as a whole: "Team learning and interprofessional

Table 2.5 Summary of McCarthy and DiGiovanni's (2017) spectrum of learning activities for interdisciplinary learning.

Low-level experience in interdisciplinary working	Mid-level experience in interdisciplinary working	High-level experience in interdisciplinary working
Classroom based Emphasis on text (books and articles, etc) Less real problem-based learning tasks	Mix of class based and clinical focused learning Moderately real simulated tasks	Use of real cases for learning and reflection Interdisciplinary presentations of case experiences Evaluations of team-based performance may be beneficial

education cannot be confined only to the classroom" (Frenk et al., 2010, p. 1944). Thus, a reasonable suggestion may be to consider whether training on mental capacity should be delivered solely to the SLT team or in collaboration with the wider professional team. Both approaches to the 'team' have different benefits.

It may be more useful to train the people who work on the unit together as a team, especially those who have to collaborate to treat service users. This team may benefit most from establishing precise roles and opinions. There is evidence of the benefit of interdisciplinary training and education as a method for reshaping health care systems and maximizing communication and collaboration between disciplines (Knab, Inzana, Cahn, & Reidy, 2017; McCarthy & DiGiovanni, 2017). The better a team works together and understands 'the process' they would need to go through in a particular situation, the more fluently they are able to address problems and challenges to reduce risk.

McCarthy and DiGiovanni describe a spectrum of learning activities for interdisciplinary learning that allows clinicians to learn with each other so that, as they continue to develop and become more experienced, they are able to learn from and about each other. These authors propose a continuum of low, mid and high levels of experience to guide teaching and interdisciplinary learning (see Table 2.5). They emphasize the value of practice-based learning where case studies can be presented virtually, simulated and then dealt with in real situations, so that teams can work together to assess and plan their management options. During planning tasks, teams should agree on the role and responsibilities of each team member and their collaborative goals, their plan and what each member of the team should accomplish within said plan, including detailing the resources required. Consequently, debriefing on the process will allow the group to consolidate their learning by discussing team communication, roles and responsibilities, equitable workload, assistance asked for or given, errors made and avoided, what went well, as well as what should change or improve.

Luff and Volkmer (2016) highlight particular approaches that can be used to explore thinking around capacity issues if there is discord within the team. Luff and Volkmer suggest the Belbin Team Roles Questionnaire (Belbin, 2010) for an established team and other more psychodynamic approaches, such as Berne's (1961) *Transactional Analysis in Psychotherapy*, or Karpman's (1968) Drama Triangle. Luff and Volkmer emphasize that it can also be useful to consider team dynamics where the team is working together effectively. This can bring to light what works well and check for subconscious collusion. Luff and Volkmer (2016) suggest some questions that may be useful to ask:

- Is there a clear team leader? Does this person always take the lead, or are there times when it is acknowledged that someone else may be better placed to take this role?

- Does everyone feel able to share their opinions? Are conversations held respectfully?

- Have cliques formed, which could lead to 'block voting' or decision making?

- Are individuals aware of their values and personal histories that may lead to bias?

When training a team, it may be useful to include discussion around key areas where conflict can arise, such as:

- What happens when there is difference of opinion as to whether an individual has decision-making capacity (pre- or post-assessment)?

- What is the best way to communicate evidence and assessment findings within the team?

- How can conflict be managed between an individual's family and the team with regards to an individual's decision-making capacity?

- How can disagreements about an individual's best interests in a given situation be managed?

It can also be useful to consider some of the key areas where conflict can arise in terms of decision-making capacity:

- Some members of the MDT deem the individual to have capacity to make a specific decision, other members disagree
- Poor communication between team members: Where a person's 'unwise' yet capacitous decision making conflicts with the team's recommendations
- Difference between family's view about capacity and that of the MDT
- Disagreement within the MDT about what constitutes best interests in a given situation
- Difference between family's view about a best interests' decision and the MDT's view.

The speech and language therapy team

Training the SLT team can facilitate an equity of knowledge, skill and service more broadly across SLTs within the Trust. The entire SLT team may wish to improve and increase their knowledge. There may be a minority of individuals with significantly more experience than others, who may be able to share knowledge and boost their colleagues' confidence. Alternatively, an SLT team can be a place of refuge to debrief and highlight areas of concern. Unfortunately, capacity issues can cause conflict between professions and it can be useful to come together within your common discipline to discuss these. These are all important and valuable reasons for training or skill development sessions within the SLT team.

It is worth mentioning, however, that both these issues – improving knowledge and supporting one another within an SLT team – highlight a broader need for policy and guidelines for the profession. Local resources, policies and guidance on the role of the SLT in decision-making capacity within the Trust can resolve many areas of concern and anxiety. New staff members appreciate pathways and guidelines. SLTs can use national and local guidelines to educate colleagues and managers on the breadth of their role. Service users deserve an equity of service and national guidelines can support SLTs in prioritizing capacity issues on their increasingly complex and diverse caseloads.

What training model will you use?

The competency-based training model is often favoured by universities. It is described as a method of structuring the learning experience and assessments so that both theoretical and practical aspects are integrated. The aim is for students to be able to demonstrate that they have achieved skills in a tangible and meaningful way (Wu, Martin, & Ni, 2017). Most often this approach targets the professional competencies outlined by a professional body such as RCSLT. As yet there are no specific competencies for SLTs around working with mental capacity. There are, however, clinical frameworks such as the Dementia Core Skills Education and Training Framework (Health Education England, 2015) that outline the essential skills and knowledge required across health and social care professionals. They outline the knowledge and duty of care for these staff when supporting people who may lack capacity. This includes guidance under section 11: Law, ethics and safeguarding in dementia care:

> "C) be able to communicate effectively about proposed treatment or care to enable people with dementia to make informed choices as far as practicable
>
> D) understand the protocols regarding consent to treatment or care for people who may lack mental capacity
>
> E) understand how 'best interests' decisions may need to be made for those lacking capacity
>
> F) know how advance directives can be used to provide information about the wishes of an individual" (p. 58).

Mastery training is another model often associated with Simulation-Based

Medical Education (SBME). The key characteristics of this model include: "(1) use of an assessment with an assessment with an established minimum passing standard, (2) definition of learning objectives aligned with the passing standard, (3) baseline assessment, (4) instruction that targets learning objectives, (5) reassessment after instruction, (6) progression to the next unit only after achievement of the passing standard, and (7) continued practice if the minimum passing standard was not achieved" (Cook et al., 2013, p. 1178). Instruction in simulation training uses simulated 'real' events and staff participate with dummies or actors. This approach is popular with medical professions, and has received some attention in the media when emergency services have used it to practise their readiness for large-scale emergencies. On a smaller scale, it has been used by psychiatrists to practise dealing with scenarios, and with trauma surgeons to ensure staff are equipped to complete surgical procedures. Simulation may be an approach that would suit the needs of allied health professionals and SLTs. SLTs are not unfamiliar with using role play as an approach in therapy, and simulation is not entirely different. Role play is certainly a useful method of safely practising communication approaches and strategies, and why should it therefore not be used successfully in practising how to support people who may lack capacity? It may be beneficial to use this in a problem-based learning approach: developing a scenario, or vignette, and inviting attendees to act out the appropriate questions and methods to support communication, with one individual taking the role of the person with communication difficulties whilst the other maintains the role of the professional assessing capacity. This method of training has been shown to improve confidence and skills in other health professionals learning how to communicate with people with aphasia (Forsgren, Hartelius, & Saldert, 2017; Saldert, Forsgren, & Hartelius, 2016;), and dementia (O'Brien et al., 2018), and may also improve confidence and skills in SLTs and other professionals training on capacity.

Training content – what will you include?

"With global platforms of knowledge on the internet, there has been a shift from memorisation of facts to location of requisite information for synthesis, analysis, and decision-making" (Frenk et al., 2010, pp. 1944-1945). Frenk et al. (2010) highlight what we all know in this day and age – that most facts can be checked on the internet. SLTs can use this wonderful facility to double-check cranial nerves, medical symptoms and the mental capacity legislation. Frenk et al. explain that "put simply, the education of health professionals in the

21st century must focus less on memorising and transmitting facts and more on promotion of the reasoning and communication skills that will enable the professional to be an effective partner, facilitator, adviser, and advocate" (2010, p. 1945). This reinforces points made earlier about developing and employing practical skills for capacity assessment. Frenk et al. suggest that the "development of the fundamental attributes of professional behaviour, identity, and values is eased by appropriate role models, team interactions, coaching, instruction, assessment, and feedback" (2010, p. 1946). This really emphasizes the need for this type of training not to be limited to a one off 'education session', but to be a broader process over a length of time. The team needs to establish a shared knowledge of the legislation and their roles (having observed and tested these roles), and then have the opportunity for mentoring and reflection to refine and hone these skills. Table 2.6 (*see over*) provides an overview of training: a pick-and-mix or flow chart of ideas that you can choose from and apply as appropriate within the department.

Reflective tools and long-term maintenance

To introduce the MCA (2005) is an important first step but, as the House of Lords post-legislative scrutiny report highlighted (in 2014), it is most important to reflect on how it is actually being used, implemented and applied in the health and social care sector. The review noted that many health and social care practitioners were struggling to apply the principles of the MCA (2005). They found that not only were practitioners not familiar enough with the Act itself but that they didn't actually know what to do in practice. This triggered a series of further recommendations, including the development of a committee to write the first NICE SCIE guidelines on decision making and mental capacity.

With the principles of reflection and critical appraisal in mind, SLTs should endeavour to include reflective practice in their clinical work. SLTs are generally good at doing this as they are often an open and reflective community of clinicians. They are likely to consider what has gone wrong and what can be improved. This includes better supporting people with communication difficulties to engage in a capacity assessment. It is not unusual to hear that an individual with aphasia, for example, who is able to engage in decision making, has been left out of important decision making because others believed that they were unable to participate. The MCA (2005) is indeed a bill of rights for our service users. We should not be afraid

Table 2.6 Overview of training ideas alongside learning objectives and activities.

Training ideas	Learning objectives	Suggested content	Practical activities	Follow-up tasks
Training days, presentations, lectures	To demonstrate an understanding of the basic principles of the MCA.	Basic summary of MCA legislation; the definition of mental capacity and the two-part assessment. This should include information on the right of an individual to make an unwise decision.	Pre-post self-rating of confidence.	Post-teaching reflection: a post-teaching assessment or case study presentation.
	To demonstrate an understanding of the two-part assessment of mental capacity.		Brainstorming or discussing the breadth of the SLT role as a group.	Assigning a mental capacity 'champion' in the department.
	To be able to consider a variety of scenarios (insert own examples) of how an assessment of decision-making capacity may be conducted.	Basic summary of the concept of best interest decision-making and advance planning. Again, drawing on the legislation itself.	Writing questions for scenarios, e.g., what can you ask to assess decision-making in regard to a dysphagia/financial/discharge decision (see a list of suggested questions in section 2 of this chapter).	Writing a departmental policy. Setting up a regular journal club or peer support group.
	To discuss the different roles an SLT may take when working with an individual who may lack capacity.	Refer to the Mental Capacity Code of Practice (2007) for more specific information on the role of the health care professional, and perhaps refer to NICE guidelines and RCSLT policy on how this should be best implemented in daily practice. These guidelines will summarize the most relevant and rigorous research.	Sharing of resources and approaches to support communication in capacity assessments.	Pooling of resources to support capacity assessments
	To demonstrate an understanding of the SLT role in best interest decision making and advance planning.		Discussion, problem solving or role playing of vignettes or scenarios (see list of vignettes and scenarios in section 2 of this chapter).	Joint sessions to increase confidence and promote consistency across the team.
	To feel more confident in working with people on issues around decision making and mental capacity.	Local guidelines may also be a useful source of information.	It is possible that your department may not have explicit guidelines as to SLT involvement in capacity assessments it may be useful to open discussions on key points such as when an SLT gets involved in a capacity assessment, any competencies that may be attached.	
	To feel more confident about when an SLT could/should become involved in a mental capacity assessment.	Ultimately, it may be recommended that this be a practical session where staff members have the opportunity to discuss and practise their skills.		
	To explore different communication support tools and techniques.		A quick test of the basic principles of the MCA and two-part assessment may be useful in gaining a clearer understanding of people's knowledge but needs to be considered carefully so as not to intimidate or alienate members of the team	
	To demonstrate an understanding of the impact of communication difficulties on mental capacity assessments and the importance of SLT involvement in this area.	Case studies designed to focus on key learning points and generate discussion.	Question and answer session.	

Training ideas	Learning objectives	Suggested content	Practical activities	Follow-up tasks
Planning days	To develop appropriate local resources to support the SLT team to deliver services to people on issues around decision-making. This may include: Developing physical resources, e.g., relevant supported communication resources A hierarchy of mentorship or supervision within the team A local policy or procedure Appropriate local referral and care pathways Training plans for SLT services, or other health and social care professionals.… New and innovative ideas.… Planning how to increase wider awareness of SLT roles and promote our involvement where applicable in mental capacity assessments e.g. considering departments to link with, use of MDT meetings, intranet, etc.	Brief review of mental capacity legislation can be a useful, confidence-boosting reminder. Asking attendees to reflect on areas of concern prior to the meeting; completing an assessment of need within the service. Although this type of exercise may equally (and usefully) be completed during the planning day. Having collated these, it can be useful to present this during the session, consequently completing tasks to prioritize need. There are numerous scientific approaches to consensus methodology, the Nominal Group Technique (Deq et al, 1974) being a favourite of the author. However, this task does not require a research methodology – this may not be clinically relevant or appropriate to get the task done. Collaborating to brainstorm and develop possible solutions is the logical next step. This may be achieved by an all-inclusive approach or group-by-group (depending on the size of the department). It is always valuable to ensure all department members feel able to contribute and that all ideas are valid. Thus, accepting and validating all contributions is key. Finally identifying important or achievable tasks with a timeline of events can act as an appropriate conclusion.	A planning day is intrinsically a practical opportunity to develop a service. Inevitably practical tasks and solutions should be interwoven in the tasks to allow full engagement. The scenario for a planning day outlined here may be tweaked and applied to specific activities including the development of a policy or a pathway. Consider different practical ways you can capture ideas and thoughts as they are generated. This should encourage contributions and engagement. Examples might include use of post-it notes and photos of generated ideas. Use of collaborative working tools such as the fishbone diagram, mindmaps, etc.	Setting up working groups to ensure identified tasks are fulfilled. Follow-up sessions or meetings to finalize plans and cascade collated information.

(Continued over)

Table 2.6 Overview of training ideas alongside learning objectives and activities. (*Continued*).

Training ideas	Learning objectives	Suggested content	Practical activities	Follow-up tasks
Developing physical resources – books, materials, web links, journal articles and other ideas (e.g., pod casts)	To provide the SLT department with accessible learning materials to support individual CPD. For SLTs in the department to have appropriate and accessible materials available to support people who may lack capacity.	It is worth stressing, as mentioned in the text, that most resources are most easily electronically available. However, it is always helpful to have a hard copy of essential guidelines and physical resources. It can be useful to keep a physical copy of the MCA (2005), the MCA Code of Practice (2007) and any other guidelines such as the forthcoming NICE SCIE guideline and the RCSLT policy. This list would of course include any local policy. Talking Mats® materials (see images in section 2) are the only communication aid or tool for which there is any research evidence. It is useful to have this available together with the appropriate local materials (e.g., images of local hospitals, wards, PEG tubes, nursing and care homes as relevant to the decision). Some if not all of the above resources are electronically available and should be either stored in a shared folder or in a list for access. Additional relevant resources will be the UK government websites where information on advance planning, power of attorney documentation and so forth is available. Some charities have excellent resources available. Many of these will not be tools that an SLT will use themselves but may need to direct people to when they ask about how to donate power of attorney etc.	Inviting teams to all contribute something: setting up a list of what everyone's top two useful things are can ensure everyone shares responsibility. Inviting an individual to act as capacity champion can ensure regular maintenance and ownership. Briefly presenting the resource to the team can improve the accessibility – making it clear and transparent. Demonstrating resources, e.g., incorporating the resources in a training session or scenario can also assist.	Annual or bi-annual maintenance of relevant resources.

Training ideas	Learning objectives	Suggested content	Practical activities	Follow-up tasks
Special interest groups and external training	For the SLT department to develop knowledge of current best practice and new research around decision-making and mental capacity.	Mental capacity is more frequently appearing on the agenda for training days and conferences The following have a particular interest: CENs e.g. London Acquired Neurology, Dementia and Mental Health of older adults (formerly Psychiatry of Old Age), Medico legal Other meetings e.g. British Aphasiology Society Therapy symposium, the RCSLT annual conference Look out for study days or presentations in MDT forums or even those directed at other disciplines. These provide useful opportunities to learn from the perspective of other disciplines and to promote the role of the SLT within the team.	Rotating attendance can be helpful. Asking people to attend in pairs to maximize discussion and reflection relevant to the department is a novel method of maximizing learning.	Presentation and sharing of information gathered within the department.

(Continued over)

Table 2.6 Overview of training ideas alongside learning objectives and activities. (*Continued*).

Training ideas	Learning objectives	Suggested content	Practical activities	Follow-up tasks
Journal clubs	To maintain an up-to-date knowledge of evidence-based care in the field of decision making and mental capacity.	The choice of article should be rotated around the group. There may be some useful and interesting texts written by SLTs that may be well worth starting with (see reference list to this chapter). The journal article should be disseminated prior to the meeting so all attendees are able to read the article. Realistic goals should be set; discussing more than one and at the most two articles is not realistic (and even this is a lot of reading to do in amongst a hectic clinical caseload). There are various methods of critiquing research literature- including the PICO method (see section 2 of this chapter for more details around critiquing methods) Realistically it may simply be worth focusing on whether a piece of research is (a) believable and (b) clinical viable in the setting you are in.	Rotating who chooses the article is an important 'task' for all attendees and to be able to search the literature is a valuable skill. Each member of the group should be encouraged to contribute. It may be worth inviting attendees to give an opinion on discrete sections so each person provides some analysis and opinion. Having said this, it can be a fine balancing act between intimidating and including team members and this may need to done sensitively and appropriately to group needs.	Discussion and opportunities to reflect on how this has been implemented in clinical practice and any challenge or barriers.

Training ideas	Learning objectives	Suggested content	Practical activities	Follow-up tasks
Workshops, knowledge cafés	For SLTs to identify their group knowledge/ opinion on a subject surrounding mental capacity.	There are many innovative methods of presenting and sharing knowledge. Workshops and knowledge cafés are two concepts that can be applied in more creative and interactive ways to develop a team's knowledge. The latter of the two is a new concept to the authors and has yet to be fully enacted in a learning setting, although it certainly shows potential. Sharing and establishing knowledge through a workshop can be a useful method of owning the knowledge in the team. For example, asking a single question of the group and then asking them to discuss, brainstorm and prioritize the answers can enable a large piece of work to be done by all members concerned. (NB. If this is being considered it is important to ensure that all team members have a sufficient understanding of 'the basics' to maximize contributions and ensure that discussions or ideas do not get ambushed by basic questions or ideas that are implausible. For example, developing a new care pathway, outcome measure or policy could be achieved in this manner. Asking the group to: "Identify and agree the pathway for a service user who is referred to the SLT service regarding concerns about mental capacity" Or "Prioritize the key roles and requirements of an SLT supporting people who around decision-making capacity in x NHS trust"		Refinement and follow-up may require further meetings, or agreement that a document will be circulated for final agreement before being adopted. Once a policy or care pathway has been developed it is important to maintain understanding and use of these documents. This can be achieved through case reflections that explicitly make reference to the care pathway or policy.

(Continued over)

Table 2.6 Overview of training ideas alongside learning objectives and activities. (*Continued*).

Training ideas	Learning objectives	Suggested content	Practical activities	Follow-up tasks
Peer support/ supervision	For SLTs to share experiences (both positive and negative) around issues related to decision-making and mental capacity in clinical practice. This may include: Case discussion Personal and professional ethics Anxieties and worries about issues such as unwise decisions where people may have chosen not to follow SLT recommendations.	Peer support and supervision is a literature unto itself. But as per these approaches a group or session should be first of all negotiated with a set of rules which may include confidentiality and mutual respect. Consequently, participants may take it in turns to share experiences, concerns and cases. Other participants may take role of listeners, supporters and supervisors.	Setting group or supervision rules is an important aspect of any type of session such as this. In addition, documenting clear actions and assigning these to a specific individual is useful, not only as a record that the meeting occurred but as a means of taking responsibility, moving things forward (and an aide memoir).	Identification and implementation of appropriate strategies or approaches into clinical practice. Resolution of roles and responsibility surrounding decision-making and mental capacity Escalation of common or key issues for resolution and discussion at a departmental level.

to take referrals and get involved. Being overwhelmed with referrals is a sure way of demonstrating that our discipline has a vital role in this area of practice.

SLTs must not rest on their laurels; they must review cases and discuss processes. They must ensure the entire team understands their role. This may include training others – colleagues in nursing and medicine, social work and other disciplines. This may also include liaising with services such as Independent Mental Capacity Advocates (IMCAs) who may be trying to represent the wishes of service users but need to understand their communication needs too. A good starting point for this may be making a link with the capacity lead in the organization.

Audit and review, annual updates and keeping ahead of the evidence may prove to be a lot of work. Yet these processes are essential to ensuring quality of care, maintaining appropriate documentation and monitoring service needs. Published audit tools can be useful; equally, establishing your own audit tool where documentation is compared to local or national guidelines for practice is useful. With this in mind, try auditing a selection of medical records retrospectively; it may be useful to assess where the SLT was involved in an issue related to decision making and mental capacity. Ask questions such as: "Is there evidence that the person was provided adequate support?" "What were these supports?" "How did the person respond?" Reviewing referral numbers and reasons for referral can also provide useful data. Comparing referral numbers year-on-year, referral sources, and outcomes (e.g., discharge destination, length of stay, etc.) can demonstrate need and activity. In the same way, analyzing risk data, near misses and complaint data can also yield valuable information on need.

Conclusion

Thus far, this chapter has provided an overview of the justification for SLTs being involved in issues related to decision-making capacity. Models of teaching and learning have been discussed and considered in relation to upskilling SLTs in the area of decision-making capacity. Finally, checklists and reflective tools have been provided and proposed to support clinicians planning to deliver training to and with SLTs.

The next section provides a set of resources to draw on, such as assessment questions, scripts and vignettes to discuss and problem solve. This complements the materials that follow in the remainder of this book. This will focus on how we as SLTs may support and train other disciplines, not forgetting the family and partners of service users who may themselves need help in decision making. In addition, Chapter 3 provides a detailed account of training sessions on the MCA and its relevance to healthcare.

Section II: Materials

Training activities

Journal article discussion

A team member selects a journal article which all attendees are invited to read prior to attending the meeting. One person may choose to briefly outline the article to the group (this is not essential). During the meeting, the attendees critique the article:

- Were the research methods sound?
- Did the theory make sense?
- What clinical implication does the article have?
- How can we change our practice to incorporate this, and should we change our practice?
- What research implications can be drawn?

There are some easily-accessible tools available for critiquing literature, including the PICO framework (Huang et al., 2006) that encourages clinicians to review the literature in the following terms:

P – What patient, problem or population is being treated/examined?

I – What is the intervention being investigated?

C – What is the comparison, control or comparator?

O – What is the outcome?

There are also other more comprehensive tools, such as the TIDieR checklist (Hoffman et al., 2014). This was developed to improve the completeness of reporting on interventions, and has subsequently been proposed as a guideline for reviewers and readers to assess intervention research. The TIDieR checklist comprises 12 questions that address areas such as what was provided, who provided it and how much was provided.

Explaining the MCA

Team members take it in turns to practise how they might explain their role in relation to the MCA to a service user (this may include an explanation of how the assessment will be carried out and why), a colleague, a superior (perhaps a medical colleague), or family member.

Team members produce a leaflet or handout on the SLT's role in mental capacity. This could ultimately be used as an informational leaflet for service users and family members and so may be produced as an accessible document.

Team members put together a web page for their department outlining their role in the same way as above. They may wish to include links to other relevant sites (e.g., government sites with information about Power of Attorney, etc.).

Presenting opportunities

Team members take it in turns to present an aspect of the MCA to their own team. This could include what this means, alongside any guidelines or policies relevant to their area of practice.

Team members take it in turns to present their own real-life cases to the team; they present the case history, the issue and the action they took. This could be used as an opportunity to share good practice, seek support and ideas for what to do next or to problem-solve what else to do, or as an opportunity to debrief.

Team members plan a presentation for their colleagues. Presenting at Grand Rounds or MDT meetings is not only a valuable learning experience for the SLT but also incredibly important in educating other disciplines on the breadth of our role. One of the most common reasons that SLTs are not involved in capacity issues is that other professionals do not fully understand our potential role and our skills.

Planning presentations could include planning training for other professionals – this is covered in more detail later in this book.

Developing resources

Team members share and develop resources (folders/electronic resources). This may include tools they prefer to use prior to the capacity assessment, including pictures, images and other resources to support communication during the assessment. Images of local hospitals, residential facilities, ethnically appropriate foods, etc., may all be useful to have handy should an individual need to participate in a capacity assessment on these topics.

Sharing resources can include sharing websites and information leaflets on future decision making, Power of Attorney, advance planning, communication books, etc.

Sharing questions can also be useful – considering how best to phrase something, how to explore someone's understanding. Making a list (see Table 2.7) and adding to it with useful examples is a good activity.

Sharing experiences

It is important to consider our own perspectives. Sharing our own opinions and feelings on a subject (what decisions we might make, how we might react, what our beliefs are on a subject) can allow us to put that aside and support people more appropriately and objectively (although arguably we can never be completely and utterly objective). Using a vignette or case study to do this can be helpful (see below for examples of case studies).

It can also be useful to share experiences more broadly: sharing a conversation, the questions we asked, the conflict that arose and how we felt about this. Do not underestimate the value of this opportunity. This is a real and important aspect of being a health professional – sharing and managing and coping. In these discussions, it is important to be respectful of others' feelings, values, beliefs and backgrounds. Providing a safe space for people to explore reactions to complex situations builds resilience and confidence as well as skills.

Role playing

Team members take it in turn (in twos or threes) in role playing scenarios – giving the opportunity to practise questions, give feedback and explore options. The case studies below can be used to guide role plays; alternatively, you may wish to generate your own from your experiences.

Questions for assessment – ideas

Team members generate questions that can be used in capacity assessments for frequent decisions faced by service users. Table 2.7 provides some example questions for capacity assessments taken from Volkmer and Luff (2016). This is not an exhaustive list by any means and just provides some ideas.

Table 2.7 NB: These questions have not been modified for anyone with receptive language difficulties or a cognitive communication difficulty. It is also important to be aware of the difference between performance capacity and judgement capacity, as discussed briefly in Chapter 1. This table does not provide an exhaustive list but may be useful during training sessions.

	Assessment questions (examples)
Consent capacity	Explain area of medical concern and recommended treatment. Advise service user of alternatives to recommended treatment. Provide information on risks of treatment and risks of choosing alternatives. *It is important to agree with the decision-maker prior to the assessment exactly what the key information is and how much the individual needs to be able to understand and retain in order to have sufficient understanding to make a decision. Although this can appear simple in practice there can be differing opinions.*
	Ask service user to recall/repeat/rephrase or summarize this information:
	What is your preference? Why do you prefer that option?
	What do you think are the pros and cons of treatment/the alternatives to the recommended treatment?
	Appelbaum (2007) suggests:
	Understanding: Tell me the problem...tell me about the treatment
	Reason: What makes this treatment option better? *Appreciation*: Why do you think your doctor has recommended this treatment?
	Communication: Have you decided...? Can you tell me your decision?
Financial	Tests of knowledge of income, assets, expenses, ability to write cheques and balance account statements, etc., as well as appreciation of how bills are paid, and consideration of financial problems and financial needs (Moberg & Pick, 2008):
	Can you tell me who you bank with and how much money you have in your accounts? Or how much goes in or out of your account on a regular basis?
	(Give service user coins/notes): Tell me which one is £1, £5, etc. If you're in a shop and you are buying a drink for X amount of money, what would you pay with and how much change would they give you? (Give service user change.) Is this the right change? What would you do if you were not given the right change?
	If you had a budget of X for one month what would you spend it on?
	(Give service user a bill): Can you tell me how much the outstanding amount is? Are there any errors on the bill?
	(Give blank cheque): Can you fill out a cheque? (Consult with OT.) Can service user use cash point, e.g., read words on screen and press correct buttons/talk to cashiers with aid if appropriate?
	What are the risks of not checking your bank statement regularly?
	What are the risks of not checking your change in a shop?
	What are the risks of not paying your credit card?
	What are the risks of not paying your bills on time?

Table 2.7 *(Continued)*

	Assessment questions (examples)
Financial *(Cont.)*	What would you do if you lost your bank card, or you noticed an error on your statement?
	Who could you ask for help? What are the risks of making purchases on the Internet? Why do you think these things would be difficult for you? Why do you think the team is concerned?
	Explain the team's concerns and recommendations and ask: Why do you think the team has recommended this?
Capacity to decide on discharge destination	What problems are you having right now? How do you think admission to a nursing home or home for the aged could help you with your condition?
	Can you think of other ways of looking after your condition?
	What could happen if you choose not to live in a nursing home or home for the aged?
	What could happen to you if you choose to live in a nursing home or home for the aged?
	The following five questions are from the Ontario Ministry of Health and Long-term Care (1997), cited by Carling- Rowland et al., 2014.
	What could be difficult when you go home?
	What do you have help with here in hospital?
	Who could you ask to help you?
	What are the risks of living on your own?
	What would happen if there were a re/burglary, etc? (Ask service user to role play this if necessary.)
	(Consult with OT/PT.) Can service user use kitchen/bathroom, etc., safely? Can service user cook and clean independently? Can service user get to shops?
	What would you do if you fell over? (Consult with OT/ PT.) What are risks of falls in home? Can service user move safely around the home?
	List some of the team's concerns and ask: Why do you think these things might be difficult for you?
	Explain the team's concerns and recommendations and ask: Why do you think the team has recommended this?
	What support would you have at home/nursing home?
	What would be good about going home/ to a nursing home?

OT = Occupational Therapist, PT = Physiotherapist

Case studies

Discussion and problem solving by using related or relevant case scenarios can be incredibly useful. What follows is a large list of cases that have been shared by other SLTs (and anonymized). Each case can be read and discussed using the following questions and considerations:

What is the decision in question?

Should and can an SLT be involved?

What would you do in this situation?

Who would you expect to be involved and with whom would you consult in this type of scenario?

What tools or resources might be useful in this scenario?

What questions might you ask the people around this person/yourself/ the person themselves?

What other information might you need to prepare for anything you would do next?

What are the issues in this scenario?

What are the cultural/ethnic/personal beliefs of this person, do you think, and how could you find out?

What is the ethical/legal issue here?

How do you feel about this situation?

Do you agree with what the SLT did in this situation; would you have done anything differently?

What do you think helped and what didn't help this situation?

Are there any other underlying issues that need to be addressed?

Suggested topics for discussion related to each case study are listed below the title.

Part 1 Acquired communication difficulties

1.1 Capacity assessment

Discharge destination

English as an additional language

The value of education prior to a capacity assessment

SLT as educator and facilitator

1.2 Capacity assessment: Non-oral feeding

Client changing their mind

Working with families

SLT as assessor

1.3 Capacity assessment: Consent to medical procedure

Positive impact of communication support on capacity assessment outcome

SLT as educator, facilitator and advocate

1.4 Capacity assessment and best interest decision: Risk feeding

Best interest does not always equate with safest option

Importance of understanding the individual and liaising with those that know him/her best

1.5 Future decision making: Advance planning

Power of Attorney

Advance directives

Conversation training with partners

Maintaining a voice in decision making

Examples of what can go wrong

1.6 Capacity assessment: Participating in research

Impact of lack of communication support on individual, family, decision outcome and relationship with staff

How to determine when SLT involvement would be useful

1.7 Capacity assessment: Marriage

Detail on SLT assessment process and input

Complexities of working with different agencies

Part 2 Capacity assessments in the acute setting

2.1 Capacity assessment: Finances

Capacity should be considered for all decisions

Individuals should be supported to engage with the decision even if they are assessed as not having capacity to make the decision

SLT as advocate

2.2 Capacity assessment: PEG placement

Consider all practicable steps to enable an individual to engage in the decision-making process

Importance of the MDT

SLT as facilitator and assessor

2.3 Capacity assessment: Discharge destination

Pictures and written words are not always helpful

Involving family in the education and assessment can be helpful

SLT as facilitator

2.4 Capacity assessment: PEG placement

Capacity is 'decision specific'

Importance of exploring consequences of decision options

Importance of identifying a client's values

SLT as assessor

Part 3 Adults with learning disability

3.1 Capacity assessment: Choosing to eat healthy foods

Use of Talking Mats©

SLT as educator and facilitator

3.2 Capacity assessment: Mealtime choices and choking risk

SLT as assessor and decision maker

Use of Talking Mats©

3.3 Capacity assessment: Marriage

Arranged marriage

MDT working

SLT as facilitator

3.4 Capacity assessment: Moving house and tenancy

MDT working

Use of objects

Positive impact of an individual being deemed to have capacity and making their own decision

3.5 Capacity assessment: Moving house

When to end SLT involvement

SLT as facilitator

3.6 Capacity assessment: Inheritance

MDT working

3.7 Capacity versus compliance with medical treatment

SLT as educator

3.8 Capacity assessment: Medical procedure (Sexually Transmitted Infection – STI screening)

MDT working

SLT assessment questions

Note: All case studies have been contributed by SLTs working with these client groups. Aspects of their clinical experiences may be reflected but all names have been changed and identifiable information omitted.

Part I Acquired communication difficulties

1.1 Capacity assessment: Facilitator – Discharge from hospital

Background

Mrs M, a lady in her mid-70s, had been admitted to the older adult wards following a fall and a diagnosed left hemisphere CVA. At this time, she was also diagnosed with moderate vascular dementia with a history of poorly-managed diabetes. Mrs M was of Greek-Cypriot descent and spoke little English. She had been living alone in her privately-owned council flat on admission. Her flat was found to be in an extremely unsanitary condition. Her two adult sons lived in Cyprus and were unable to provide any regular support.

Mrs M remained on the inpatient ward for six months' rehabilitation. During this time, she made some improvements but required ongoing support with communication, medication monitoring and adherence, continence and other activities of daily living. The team recommended a long-term living facility equipped to support her complex medical needs alongside ongoing community rehabilitation. The team had been expressing some concerns about her decision making on the ward based on some risk-taking behaviour, and her ongoing poor diabetes self-management (even with lengthy education and support with a Greek interpreter and the SLT involved).

Action

A capacity assessment was conducted in which the team explained the aim and plan for assessment using an interpreter and the SLT to support her communication. The OT supported Mrs M in a home visit to her flat to see the condition of the accommodation, taking photos whilst there. The team provided a rationale for the team recommendations – using photos of home, and the participant receiving assistance during ADLs. Supported conversation was used during the conversation (using gesture, images, written single words and a Talking Mat (see Figure 2.2 for an example of a Talking Mat). The OT also supported Mrs M to visit a number of other long-term living facilities equipped to support her needs. Mrs M discussed the pros and cons of both living situations using the Talking Mats© tool to aid discussion.

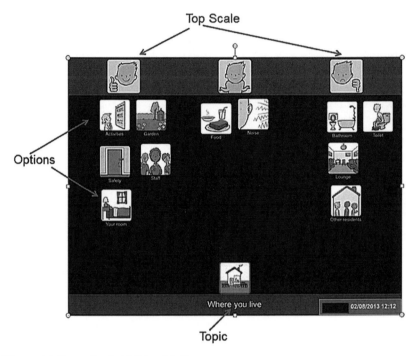

Figure 2.2 Example of a Talking Mat©.

Outcome

In discussion with the social worker and the SLT, Mrs M demonstrated an understanding of the recommendations, and was able to recall the discussion related to this, including the visits. She demonstrated capacity and expressed a decision to follow the team recommendations even though this wasn't her initial preference. It was formally agreed that the team would recommend that staff in the supported accommodation review her living situation in 6–12 months' time. To this end, her sons proposed they would pay for their mother's accommodation so she would be able to retain the flat, at which time they would revisit the decision. The team advised that the situation may not have changed to the point that she would be able to live independently at this time. Mrs M's sons stated that their mother was stubbornly independent and needed to be given this opportunity to return home in the future.

1.2 Capacity assessment: Assessor – Swallowing

Background

Mr S had been diagnosed with Motor Neurone Disease two-and-a-half years ago. He was aged 55 and presented with moderate dysphagia and dysarthria alongside significant weight loss. Mr S was a lawyer by background and lived with his wife and two adult children. He described himself as headstrong and independent.

A videofluoroscopy showed significant risk of aspiration. Alongside this Mr S reported discomfort and displeasure when eating and drinking. Mr S was provided with information on alternative feeding during a home visit; the videofluoroscopy X-ray (X-ray of his swallow) was shown to him and used to explain the pros and cons of oral versus non-oral feeding. The process of referring for a percutaneous endoscopic gastroscopy (PEG) (to the specialist medical and nursing teams) and other non-oral intake options was described. Pictorial resources (Figure 2.3) were used to demonstrate how the non-oral feeding works and illustrate the appearance of the PEG. Mr S expressed interest in alternative feeding and consented to a referral in this session. Later, his wife worriedly telephoned to report he had changed his mind.

Action

The SLT returned to assess Mr S's decision making in person as he could not discuss the issue by phone due to his dysarthria. She explained the rationale for the assessment. Mr S is aware of the MCA legislation. The SLT revisited the information provided at the previous session. Mr S was able to demonstrate his understanding and retention of the information provided at the previous session. He was able to write down a list of reasons for his decision for the SLP and clearly explain why he had changed his mind.

Outcome

Mr S and the SLT agreed that he has the right to change his mind. They agreed that they will need to support his wife in this decision. As a result, the same discussion was held with the wife present. Following this discussion, the SLT and the GP revisited the decision with Mr and Mrs S on a number of occasions but Mr S continued to demonstrate good rationale and Mrs S reported feeling more comfortable with his decision after a number of meetings.

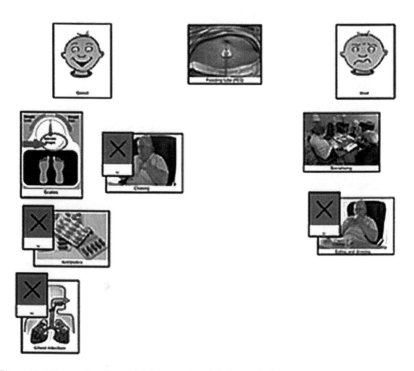

Figure 2.3 Example of how the Supporting Adults with Communication Impairment to make Decisions, ref '06' resource written by Allen & Bryer, 2014, can be used in discussions about non-oral feeding options (reproduced by permission of Black Sheep Press Ltd). This can be accessed at https://www.blacksheeppress.co.uk/product/supporting-adults-communication-impairment/.

1.3 Capacity assessment: Facilitator/advocate – Consenting to medical procedure

Background

Mr B, a gentleman of 57 years, was admitted to the rehabilitation ward with a stroke-related aphasia (moderate–severe) and some cognitive difficulties (attention, planning, memory). He also presented with some physical difficulties including poor balance and concerns that he may have a visual field impairment. He had previously had a cataract operation in his right eye and also presented with diabetes. Mr B lived alone, had no family and was of West Indian heritage. He would often become aggressive and anxious; shouting at and threatening staff in the evenings. He was also experiencing difficulties moving about the ward at night, tripping and nearly falling. Staff were concerned about his mental state and ability to live independently. After further discussion supported by the SLT it became apparent that he believed people were observing him. He reported late family members standing outside his door and at the bottom of his bed. These experiences were likely a combination of visual difficulties and his spiritual beliefs. Staff recommended a second cataract operation.

Action

Staff felt concerned that Mr B would not have the capacity to consent to a cataract operation due to his day-to-day memory difficulties and some concerns around decision making on the ward. The team recommended the SLT attend the appointment with ophthalmology in order to ensure all possible assistance would be available to support Mr B's communication. Prior to this appointment the SLT reviewed Mr B's communication skills. The SLT discussed plans to attend the appointment and provided large font appointment information about the details of the appointment. Mr B agreed that the ophthalmologist would benefit from advice around his own communication and jointly drafted an advice sheet with the SLT to give to the staff there.

The SLT attended the appointment with Mr B, where the ophthalmologist recommended a cataract operation. The SLT developed a large, accessible information sheet using information given by the ophthalmologist. The SLT discussed the information with Mr B, who consequently voiced some concerns about aftercare. The SLT attended the pre-op appointment where Mr B was able to demonstrate his understanding and ask planned questions without prompting from the SLT.

Outcome

Mr B demonstrated he could retain, recall, and weigh up all information given and express his decision to consent to the operation. He was also able to voice his preferences around managing his own aftercare, based on his previous experiences prior to this stroke.

1.4 Capacity assessment and best interest decision: Modified consistencies vs 'normal' food and drink

Background

Mr J, an 87-year-old, had been diagnosed with Parkinson's disease 26 years ago. He had also presented with a dementia, likely a Parkinson's dementia, and was awaiting a review with his consultant to confirm this. Mr J lived at home with his wife and had previously owned his own business in the construction industry. He had three adult children who lived nearby. He was seen by the SLT for a swallow review on a background of worsening dysphagia over the last three years. The SLT felt concerned that he was likely aspirating on thin fluids. He had no history of chest infections or choking, although weight loss was a concern. The SLT recommended syrup thick fluids and a mince-mashed diet. A videofluoroscopy examination confirmed these concerns and recommendations. On a review visit Mr J's wife reported he had been refusing thickened fluids at home and requesting normal foods.

Action

Even with communication supports a capacity assessment demonstrated that Mr J was unable to demonstrate an understanding of the risks around aspiration. The SLT discussed the issues at length with Mr J's wife. She reported that Mr J has made "unwise decisions" throughout his life, often including not following medical advice. He had always been fussy about his food preferences and still enjoyed the food he did like (pies, sausages and other traditional foods). She felt he considered food a core part of his quality of life. In Mrs J's opinion, Mr J would prefer not to follow the SLT recommendations.

The SLT discussed the issues further with the GP and Mr J's wife. They discussed Mr J's previous beliefs and values. They discussed the risk of aspiration, dehydration and concerns around weight loss.

Outcome

They agreed that it is currently in Mr J's best interest (as per his preference) to eat and drink what he wished and thus potentially gain or at least maintain his weight (alongside a re-referral to the dietitian). It was agreed that this should be reviewed regularly should anything change in the future.

1.5 Future decision making: Advance planning

Background

Mr S was diagnosed with Primary Progressive Aphasia (the language-led frontotemporal dementia) in his late 50s. He had been living with the diagnosis for three years when he was referred to speech and language therapy. Mr S had been a history lecturer when he was first diagnosed and had since retired. He lived with his wife and two teenage children. Mr and Mrs S had already donated Power of Attorney to one another for health and welfare decisions and personal affairs just prior to his diagnosis.

Action

Mr S felt generally anxious about the future. One of his concerns was that his family would find it difficult to make decisions related to his end-of-life care. He felt keenly that he wanted to support them, and retain his voice in his own care for as long as possible. The SLT suggested he write an advance directive, which he did independently outside of the session. He was also working on a communication book in therapy and he decided to include a large section in the book on future decision making. This included information on his advance directive as well as other preferences related to his day-to-day care.

As his language deteriorated, Mr S continued to express concerns about being involved where possible with future decisions. The SLT suggested that as part of the advice she had been giving to Mr S's wife, working on conversation training may also be useful. The SLT used the Better Conversations with PPA (BCPPA, Volkmer et al., forthcoming) training program to start the communication training. The final session focused on planning for future changes in communication. Having reflected on the barriers and facilitators in conversation, Mr S and his wife were able to reflect on how strategies may continue to enable him to participate in conversations. This discussion also focused on exactly how Mr S's communication book should and could be used in future conversations.

1.6 Capacity assessment: Participating in research

Background

Mrs V was a 71-year-old aphasic service user on the stroke ward. She had a supportive husband who visited her most days. Mrs V had previously worked as a dinner lady in the local school and had only recently retired. She remained proactive in the local community and nearby church. Volunteering at a local day centre for older adults had been a weekly routine for her and her husband. Mrs V had a diagnosis of a stroke, her sisters, her mother and her aunts had all also had a stroke in the past. Mrs V had recovered quickly and the medical registrar suggested she might like to participate in a research study.

Action

Mrs V was approached by one of the research students in the study without advance notice being given to her husband. The student reported to his consultant that the lady had been very 'difficult' and had refused to participate in the study. The consultant told the student not to bother asking again. The husband later lodged a complaint with the nursing staff that his wife had been consulted about some research and neither of them knew what was going on. He approached the nursing staff again a week later asking for more information – this was raised in the team meeting.

The SLT suggested it might be helpful to the consultant and the research student if she attend the meeting. The consultant declined the offer. Mrs V raised some questions about the research to the SLT in her therapy session, stating she was keen to help wherever she could. Mrs V stated she wanted to do the research but hadn't understood what the researcher was saying and had wanted her husband to be present for the meeting.

The SLT pursued the discussion with the consultant with no further success. Some weeks later, the student researcher returned without informing the SLT or the husband, and this time reported he had consented Mrs V to the study.

Outcome

Mrs V's husband made a complaint to the hospital and Mrs V was withdrawn from the study.

1.7 Capacity assessment: Facilitator – Marriage

Background

An old-age psychiatrist referred a gentleman, P, with post-stroke aphasia in his mid-60s, to SLT asking for support with a capacity assessment. P and his partner, J, had been together for 20 years and had lived together since his stroke. They had been to the registry office two months previously to give notice of marriage. This had been declined as the registrar had some concerns that P was not able to consent to the marriage as he was unable to answer their questions. P and J had tried to gain support from their local MPs but had not received an adequate response. Following this they approached P's GP, who referred him to the local old-age psychiatry team for a mental capacity assessment (MCA).

Prior to and during the assessments with P, the SLT wanted to ensure she was following the correct procedures with regard to supporting a capacity assessment. She spoke with the Trust's mental capacity advisor to confirm that she was fulfilling her role appropriately. She did some reading on the MCA and marriage. Along with its key principles it states "that all practicable steps must be taken to help the person to make a decision". Another statement of relevance to this case was that "nothing in this Act permits a decision on any of the following matters to be made on behalf of a person - (a) consenting to marriage or a civil partnership...". On questioning whether an MCA therefore should be embarked upon in this instance she read further, in the context of mental capacity and learning disability, that "although a person cannot make a decision about marriage on another's behalf, the principles of the Act can be used to determine whether or not a person with a learning disability who is to be or has been forced into marriage has the capacity to give informed consent" (Forced Marriage and Learning Disabilities: Multi-Agency Practice Guidelines, HM Government). Following this, "If the person lacks the capacity to consent to the marriage, one course of action is for the local authority to make an application to the Court of Protection for declarations and orders."

Knowing then that it would be appropriate to facilitate an MCA the SLT prepared to facilitate P's communication during the assessment.

Action

The SLT saw P for four assessment sessions, using formal and informal assessment to develop a communication profile. From a basic communication screen, she saw that P's receptive language was significantly stronger than his expressive language, which was also impacted by verbal dyspraxia. He had minimal verbal output which mainly consisted of automatic phrases. P's verbal yes/no consistency was poor, as he often spoke using automatic phrases instead of 'yes' or 'no'. On trialling a yes/no chart, P appeared confused by pointing to yes or no and did not show consistency. He was however able to follow three-step instructions. On reading comprehension assessment, he performed well and was able to consistently match single written words to pictures by pointing. The SLT also performed some informal assessment at P's house, with his partner present, observing how they communicated. They appeared to do a lot of communication practice together and P was observed to be able to point to specific written words in books when J read aloud. It was also useful to see P at home because he could become distressed at new forms of assessment or when in unfamiliar places, but performed much better when relaxed and performing a familiar task.

In order to determine whether P could understand, retain, weigh up and communicate whether he wanted to marry J, the HM Government's guidelines state these possible questions as examples:

- What is a husband/wife?

- What is a marriage?

- What is different about being married or unmarried?

After liaison with the psychiatrist, a list of relevant questions was drawn up which aimed to determine whether P fully understood what marriage was. As marriage does not have clear 'risks' or 'benefits', the weighing-up questions were difficult. However, as the team had gathered background information on the case, they were able to include some questions such as, "How might your family feel if you get married?", which could give an insight to whether P could weigh up the risks, i.e., that his family might be upset.

A list of 10 questions was drawn up; these were provided in the format deemed most appropriate for P following the SLT assessment, where his strengths had been in verbal and written comprehension. For the majority of the questions, the answer was known, e.g., the team knew that P and J had been together for 20 years.

Example of a multiple-choice question that P was asked:

If you do get married how might your family feel?

☐ be unhappy   ☐no change   ☐ be happy

The assessment was arranged for 10am at P's local hospital as this was reported to be a good time of day for him.

Outcome

Two psychiatrists led the assessment with the SLT facilitating communication. J accompanied P but was asked to leave the room during the assessment. P was introduced to the questions and asked to point to his choice of answer out of the three options for each question. P answered eight of the ten questions 'correctly'. J was subsequently asked to come in and the psychiatrists informally assessed P's interactions with her. A discussion was held amongst the three professionals following the assessment and P was deemed to have demonstrated capacity to make the decision to get married.

Yet despite the decision made by the psychiatrists that P demonstrated the capacity to make the decision to marry, on their return to the registry office to give notice of marriage with the psychiatrists' report, P and J were again declined. The registrar stated that this was because P would still need to be able to demonstrate an ability to answer the questions required in a giving notice meeting (for example, "What is your full name?", "What is the full name of your partner?"). The SLT and the registrar discussed P's communication and his aphasia. It was explained that P would require reasonable adjustments in order for him to access the service of marriage, as per the Equality Act 2010. Unfortunately, the registry office declined to make these adjustments as they felt the adjustments needed (for example, providing multiple choice answers) contradicted current marriage law and would be leading P towards a particular decision.

Outcome

The couple have taken the issues forward with The Equality and Human Rights Commission, which provides advice on disability discrimination.

Part II The acute setting

2.1 Capacity assessment: Finances

Background

B had been admitted to hospital following a fall. He had previously sustained a traumatic brain injury as a result of a similar fall six months previously which had left him with a moderate dysarthria and further mobility problems. He also had a 'known' cognitive impairment but no formal diagnosis of dementia. During his admission B had repeated chest infections and, when unwell, became delirious and found it more difficult to follow conversation and retain information. During his admission B's wife passed away at home. At this point B had an active delirium. He became immediately upset and agitated by the information. The social worker visited on multiple occasions to discuss his wife's funeral arrangements as she had not indicated any wishes or made any plans. Despite the involvement of friends and attempts to provide simplified information B was too upset and agitated to engage in any conversation about the funeral. At times, he refused to believe she had passed away and at other points was too agitated to engage at all. A decision needed to be made and on the social worker's assessment it was determined that B did not have capacity to make decisions about his wife's funeral. Arrangements were then made by the local authority. At this point it appeared that B had lost control or influence over his wife's funeral.

Action

The SLT worked with B and a member of the old-age psychiatry team who B knew and trusted to talk through what had happened and to help him engage in what was going to happen. B expressed concerns that he didn't have a suit to wear to the funeral and that he wanted to buy everyone a drink who attended the funeral. Over time B's delirium and emotional state improved and he was able to engage further in these conversations. Through supported conversation and the use of options and closed questions to keep B on topic, he was able to identify the suit he wanted to wear and the SLT ensured that the social worker retrieved it from his home. This immediately made B calmer on the ward. He forgot, at times, that the issue had been addressed but only needed to be shown the suit to feel reassured. Issues and options around paying for food/drink at the funeral were discussed with the SLT and written down to assist B in recalling the pros and cons of each option as he saw it. A capacity assessment was completed by the social worker with the SLT facilitating. It was agreed that B demonstrated capacity to make a decision about spending money on food, drink and flowers at the funeral.

Outcome

B attended his wife's funeral in the suit he wanted to wear and ensured that everyone who was there had a drink that he had bought for them. It was of course a very sad occasion, but on returning to the ward B repeatedly reflected how pleased he was that he had been able to buy their friends a drink.

2.2 Capacity assessment: PEG placement

Background

E, a 78-year-old woman, had recently had a stroke that resulted in a number of impairments including a moderate expressive and receptive aphasia, a moderate oropharyngeal dysphagia and right-sided hemiplegia. She had been discharged to a nursing home with recommendations to take syrup thick fluids and a fork-mashed diet. She was readmitted to hospital three weeks following discharge with dehydration, lethargy and apparent refusal or inability to eat/drink. E's family were very upset about the situation. One of her daughters believed she was no longer able to swallow. Her son thought she was 'trying to die' because she did not want to be in a nursing home.

Action

The SLT attempted to assess E's swallow on multiple occasions with and without family present. On most occasions she closed her eyes, clamped her mouth shut and turned away, regardless of the food being offered. Occasionally she would answer yes/no to questions but this was found not to be consistent even about basic biographical information. Pictures and Talking Mats© were used in an attempt to gain an understanding of E's views and wishes but she rarely engaged and it became clear that yes/no questions were the most successful in eliciting a response from her. The SLT contacted the old-age psychiatry team with the aim of determining if E might be depressed, and whether this was contributing to her apparent refusal to eat/drink and overall lack of engagement. Again, limited information was gleaned from E who answered questions about whether she wanted to die with both 'yes' and 'no' during the same conversation. The team felt there was sufficient evidence to suggest E was depressed. A capacity assessment was completed with the medical team, around nasogastric (NG) tube placement. E's responses to questions remained inconsistent and she did not demonstrate an ability to make a decision about NG tube placement. A decision involving her family was made in her best interest.

An NG tube was placed for a trial period of three weeks. The aim was to provide E with nutrition, hydration and antidepressants with the hope that this would improve her ability to engage in conversation and then discuss oral and, if necessary, non-oral feeding options further. Consideration was given to E's location on the ward with an attempt to give her a window view as her family reported that losing her garden was one of the most upsetting consequences of her move to the nursing home. Attempts were also made to engage E with food and drink cooked by her family or bought from her favourite takeaway.

Outcome

Unfortunately, after three weeks there was no improvement in E's presentation.

A capacity assessment was completed around percutaneous endoscopic gastrostomy (PEG) placement. Despite education sessions and attempts to involve her daughter E did not engage in the assessment. A decision was made in her best interest to have a PEG placed. The family revisited the decision about discharge to home and a trial period with family taking turns to stay with their mother alongside a care package was agreed. It was agreed that food/drink would continue to be offered to E and should circumstances change E could be involved in a future decision about removing the PEG.

2.3 Capacity assessment: Discharge destination

Background

D, a 72-year-old lady with a mixed vascular and Alzheimer's dementia, had been admitted to hospital following a fall at home. She was subsequently diagnosed with a urinary tract infection (UTI). D was increasingly frail and was assessed as having multiple care needs upon discharge. The social worker involved in her care referred to the SLT to support a capacity assessment around discharge destination, as she had previously found that the use of some of the SLT's written and pictorial resources had been helpful in guiding conversation and enabling other clients to demonstrate their understanding of the issues.

Action

The SLT had not previously met D and so agreed with the social worker that she would carry out at least two sessions prior to the capacity assessment to gather information and assess the best way to support D's communication. On assessment it became clear that written and pictorial information was distracting to D and she was unable to relate this to the topic of conversation. The SLT introduced the issue of discharge destination and talked through the options outlined by the social worker. D lost track of the conversation quickly but with a quiet environment and verbal prompting was able to recall the key information. The SLT asked D if she would like anyone involved in helping her to make a decision. D's son lived with her and she was very keen to have his involvement. He was briefed on the decision and on the aim of establishing his mother's views and therefore the need to be neutral and non-leading unless she asked for his opinion. He was told that his mother's capacity to make this decision would be assessed the following week. Education sessions were carried out with the SLT and D's son through the week. It was clear that

D was more motivated to engage in discussion with her son and was at ease with his prompting style.

Outcome

At D's request her son was present at the capacity assessment. D clearly demonstrated an understanding of the decision and options and was able to weigh her options and communicate her decision. D was deemed to have capacity to make the decision and was discharged home with a package of care.

2.4 Capacity assessor: PEG placement

Background

Y, a 70-year-old man, was admitted to hospital with worsening dysarthria. Five years prior to admission he had a stroke which left him with a moderate mixed dysarthria and mild weakness in his right arm and leg. Y had no known family. He had lived in charity-run sheltered accommodation for 20 years and was a very valued member of their community. Y was unable to read and write and it was thought he likely had an undiagnosed learning disability. On this admission Y was diagnosed with bilateral cortical infarcts and pseudo bulbar palsy. He presented with severe oropharyngeal dysphagia. A videofluoroscopy (swallowing X-ray) was performed and aspiration (food/fluid passing the vocal cords towards the lungs) was seen to occur on all consistencies of food and drink. The options for managing his swallowing difficulty and eating and drinking were discussed with Y and he agreed to remaining nil by mouth for the time being, demonstrating capacity to make this decision. It was agreed to commence a programme of swallow trials and therapy over a three-week period with the aim of improving the comfort and safety of his swallow. Unfortunately, on repeat videofluoroscopy there had been no meaningful change. Y found eating and drinking uncomfortable but reported that he wanted to continue having small amounts of water and a puree dessert in the evening, accepting any risk that accompanied this. A capacity assessment was carried out by the SLT and Y demonstrated capacity to make this decision. Strategies were discussed and implemented to maximize the safety of his oral intake. During his admission, he maintained these preferences and did not seek to eat or drink any more. A PEG was suggested, by the consultant looking after Y, as a relatively safe long-term solution essential for meeting Y's nutritional requirements and prolonging his life.

Action

The SLT carried out assessments looking at how best to support Y's understanding. Pictures had been identified as useful in helping Y follow a conversation about new information but he became overwhelmed and confused if there were too many and worked best with a maximum of four pictures during a conversation. Because of his dysarthria anything beyond a one-word response was difficult to comprehend, even by a familiar listener. The SLT discussed with the gastroenterologist and consultant the level of understanding required to make the decision. Following this, the SLT undertook four education sessions to work on Y's understanding of key points related to the procedure and the risks/benefits attached to each of these. Along with all of the generic risks/benefits associated with having a PEG it was clear that one of the most important for Y would be whether a PEG meant he would have to leave his home and community of the last 20 years. In discussion with Y he clearly indicated that he valued being back with his friends even for a short while more than prolonging his life. Therefore, alongside the education sessions for Y, the SLT worked with the social worker to discuss his situation with the manager of the sheltered accommodation. The manager had reservations and initially it was not clear that Y would be accepted back if he had a PEG and associated care needs. The manager's concerns were discussed and ways to support Y and the home were provisionally arranged.

Outcome

A capacity assessment was carried out by the registrar and facilitated by the SLT. Although regular education sessions had been carried out with Y he struggled to recall the complex and new information and was becoming increasingly anxious about having an operation and about going home. Despite support Y was assessed as not having capacity to make a decision about PEG insertion. (NB: Retention is not required between sessions only for time required to make the decision.) A best interests meeting was held and Y's preferences to continue eating just very small amounts and to go home were considered. Y had a PEG placed and went home with support from community services.

Part III: Adults with learning disability

The following case examples have been shared by SLTs working with adults with learning disabilities. Our thanks to Karen Bamford, Clinical Lead SLT in the

Learning Disabilities Service, Birmingham Community Healthcare Trust and her team for sharing these examples. All the examples described below have been anonymized and are based on the team's experiences in clinical practice.

3.1 Capacity assessment: Facilitator – Choosing and eating healthy foods

Background

A 32-year-old gentleman, H, was referred to the SLT service by the dietician to assess whether he had capacity to choose and eat healthy food. The dietician wanted to find out whether H was able to understand the consequence of being overweight and had the ability to choose healthy foods, as it was causing several health issues that were impacting his treatment and overall management.

H had mild learning disability. He lived at home with his family and attended a day centre five days per week. H was mobile and was able to access local shops independently in the community. When he went to the local shops he usually chose crisps, drinks, chocolates and takeaways like fish and chips, donner meat, kebabs, etc. H had two–three key word level understanding and his verbal expression was predominantly in single words and short phrases.

Action

The SLT visited H at home to gather information on his eating habits/routine from his family. His mother informed the SLT that H helped himself to whatever food was available and there were no set timings to when or what he ate. When eating a meal with the family, he continued to eat without realizing that he had had enough. He occasionally vomited after a big meal. At the day centre, he had a main meal with pudding, and had money to buy additional fizzy drinks, chocolate and crisps from the canteen. A joint visit was arranged with the dietician to establish a baseline. A series of simple questions were formulated to use as a basis in the capacity to consent assessment. The SLT used Talking Mats© approach (see Figure 2.4), pictures and symbols to find out H's likes/preferences and dislikes with foods. He expressed a preference towards the unhealthy foods.

The SLT provided information to H by talking about what happened when he chose healthy foods and when he consumed unhealthy food using a range of relevant pictures and symbol resources. The SLT simplified dietetic advice regarding eating meals in small portion sizes and at set times. She talked about the consequences of being overweight, for example low energy levels, feeling lethargic, breathing difficulties, walking difficulty, etc. They also talked about long-term health implications such as diabetes and stroke.

At a follow-up session, foods were further classified into healthy and unhealthy food choices. H was able to identify the majority of the healthy foods such as fruits, vegetables, sandwiches in brown bread, cheese, milk, fish, yoghurt and water in comparison to unhealthy foods such as biscuits, cakes, chocolates, oily and fried food. In fact, he said "five portions", "fruit", "healthy". The SLT facilitated the session by simplifying the questions asked by the dietician. For example, when asked "What would help you to lose weight?", H said "eating less", "choosing healthy foods", "exercise". "How does it feel after you have eaten a large portion of food?" H said "sick". "What will happen when you continue to eat unhealthy foods?" H said, "high cholesterol", "heart problem", "health problems". H verbally agreed to choose healthy foods and follow the dietician's advice on his weight management.

Outcome

Following this assessment, it was established by the decision maker (dietician) that H had the capacity to choose and eat healthy foods. He was aware of the long-term consequences. In order for H to follow dietetic advice, the SLT agreed to adapt the information booklet into an accessible format with pictures and easy-to-read text. A visual planner was also created for H to follow set mealtimes and portion sizes with healthy food options as a reminder.

3.2 Capacity: Assessor and decision maker – Mealtime choices and choking risk

Background

A referral was received by the learning disability SLT team for E, an 87-year-old lady who had lived at her nursing home for five years. The referral was made by the home manager following a Care Quality Commission (CQC) inspection where E was observed to be refusing modified food and was requesting a more normal diet. E had a diagnosis of mild/moderate learning disability and frailty. She also had had a stroke resulting in a right-sided hemiparesis and dysphagia and was currently recommended Texture D (pre-mashed) foods and regular

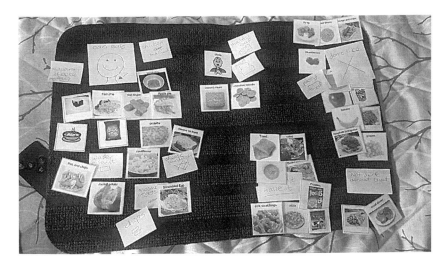

Figure 2.4 Example of a Talking Mat© layout used with H.

drinks. E had no dentition and didn't wear dentures. The home manager stated that E had experienced a few occasions of what she called 'choking' in the past.

Action

The SLT visited the nursing home on three separate occasions. The SLT first reviewed E's eating and drinking recommendations. E understood the reason for these visits and consented to the assessments taking place. E understood the information relevant to the decision. She knew the meals she had each day, she named her favourite foods and talked about safe textures, and foods that she used to have but couldn't have now. When asked why foods needed to be soft she reported that she used to choke with hard foods and had to stop having them. E was able to say how some of the foods she liked could be made soft, including making cake soft by adding custard. E stated that she doesn't choke now because the food is soft and that she wouldn't want hard foods now.

Assessment of E's decision making regarding what she ate was completed with the help of a Talking Mat©. A range of food symbols was offered with top scales of 'I can eat', 'Make me cough', 'Don't like', 'I don't have it' and 'I'm not sure'. E selected and placed food symbols for each of these scales in line with her current eating skills and her knowledge of risk of coughing and choking.

She discussed with the SLT many of the symbols she selected (e.g., that she can eat soft snacks, and has cauliflower mashed). E retained the information relevant to the decision. She accurately recalled and discussed information from previous visits with the SLT. E used or weighed the information as part of the process of making a decision. E talked about foods that she could have (soft foods, and staff supporting her with mashing and cutting up foods) and foods she cannot have (foods that are hard, foods she used to choke on, foods she has stopped having and wouldn't want to eat now). E communicated her decision, confirming her favourite foods and communicating the risks of having foods that are hard to eat.

Outcome

E demonstrated capacity to make a decision about what she ate. The SLT advised that Texture D (pre-mashed) foods were preferable for E and that Texture E (fork mashable) foods were to be provided if E requested them.

3.3 Capacity assessment: Facilitator – Marriage

Legislative background

The MCA Code of Practice (2007) is clear about the decisions which are excluded from anyone making a decision on someone else's behalf. These include decisions concerning family relationships (Section 27). This means that no-one else may make a decision on someone's behalf involving consenting to marriage or a civil partnership or sexual relations. Whilst no-one may make a decision regarding consenting to a marriage where someone lacks capacity to consent, it may be that an assessment of decision-making capacity is required to establish whether the individual has the capacity to consent to the decision themselves. Such a case is described below.

General background

A gentleman was referred to the SLT service to facilitate a capacity to consent assessment regarding marriage. He was in his 30s, with a moderate learning disability, depression and forensic needs and lived at home with his family. His mother had discussed with his community nurse about arranging a marriage for her son with a lady who lived in Pakistan. His community nurse started with the presumption that the gentleman had capacity to make a decision regarding marriage but felt that, due to his impairment in the functioning of his mind or brain (stage 1), that this impairment may mean that he was unable to make a specific decision and that they needed (stage 2) to make an assessment of his capacity to consent in this area using all practical and appropriate support.

Actions

The social worker acted as the decision maker in this case, and the SLT facilitated communication during the assessment. Marriage is defined in the *Oxford English Dictionary* as "The legally or formally recognized union of two people as partners in a personal relationship". This is an individual union which establishes rights and obligations between spouses and their wider networks. A meeting was held between the allocated social worker and SLT to establish the information relevant to marriage and develop a series of simple questions to use as a basis in the capacity to consent assessment.

The SLT then created a series of related photo and symbol resources in order to focus the gentleman to the relevant information, e.g., culturally relevant weddings, relationship-based symbols and photographs. The social worker and SLT then met with the gentleman and, after building rapport with him, were able to carry out the capacity to consent assessment focusing on:

1. Understanding the information relevant to the decision; that in his case his marriage would be between him and a woman, being able to define what marriage would mean to him, what a wedding would be for him.

2. Retain the information relevant to the decision.

3. Use or weigh-up the information relevant to the decision; that in his case what could the good things be about getting married, what could be bad things be about getting married.

4. Communicate his decision.

Outcome

Following this assessment, it was established by the decision maker that, having used all practical means, the gentleman lacked capacity to consent in the area of marriage. The SLT then supported the gentleman to understand the outcome of the assessment and what that meant for him, in an accessible format.

3.4 Capacity assessment: Joint assessment – Moving house and tenancy

Background

When considering taking on responsibilities such as independent living it is important to ensure that individuals who sign documents, such as tenancy agreements, understand the implications of contracts and the possible consequences of taking on these responsibilities. One such case was a lady with a moderate learning disability who lived in a communal residential home. She decided that she would like to live independently (on her own) with care hours. It was established that this could be achieved by finding an appropriate privately-rented flat with care hours from a care provider. For this to proceed the lady needed to be able to legally sign a tenancy agreement, demonstrating capacity to consent to the conditions on the tenancy. The lady in question occasionally showed signs of challenging behaviour including property damage. Those involved with her current care felt concerned about the implications of her behaviour and property damage in a rental flat.

Action

A capacity to consent assessment took place together with her social worker, using a range of reasonable means of communication such as objects and drawings developed by her SLT. In terms of understanding the relevant information in the area of tenancy, this lady could identify vocabulary such as 'rent', 'lord' (a shortened version of landlord due to speech sound difficulties), 'no argue'. She was able to identify possible consequences of not following her tenancy agreement such as 'put you in court', 'tells you to go away'. In addition to this piece of work objects such as those in Figure 2.5 were used to discuss the pros and cons of a tenancy agreement. These were used to identify who is responsible for household objects if they get broken.

It was agreed that the specific elements of this lady's and her private landlord's tenancy were put into an easy-to-read format that were agreed and signed together.

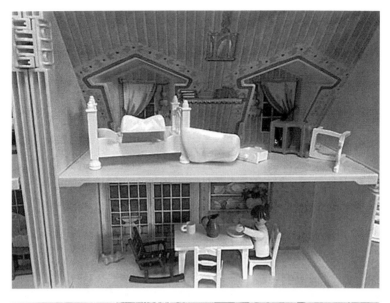

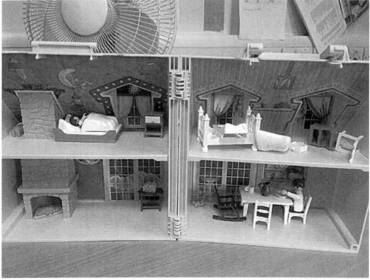

Figure 2.5 Objects to support discussion.

Outcome

This lady has now lived independently for four years, where she has held and complied with a tenancy agreement. In addition to this, there has been a marked reduction in challenging behaviour.

3.5 Capacity assessment: Facilitator – Moving house

Background

This case involved a lady with a diagnosis of Down Syndrome, a profound and multiple learning disability, and a severe communication impairment (meaning she understood one key word at a time based on information within the here and now). Her understanding was based on familiar words and topics that she had experience of. She had always lived within her family home with her mother and father. Her mother had historically provided the majority of her care and had recently passed away. Whilst her elderly father was supportive in continuing to live with his daughter, there were questions regarding his ability to provide a sufficient level of care for her.

Action

Due to the changes in this lady's circumstances, it had been agreed by social services that she would temporarily move to respite care whilst permanent care was arranged. This review included a formal capacity assessment led by the social worker and facilitated by the SLT. The lady in question showed a clear preference for living with her father, though she had no experience of living anywhere else but the family home and was not able to consider what living in other accommodation and with other care requirements would be like. In terms of reasonable means of communication, she was not able to use pictures to help her communicate issues outside of the here and now. When discussing the issues at hand, the lady was unable to identify where she currently lived, what care needs she had, who would provide her help and what her accommodation options were.

Outcome

It was deemed that SLT could not provide further facilitation of her communication due to her limitations and that she lacked capacity to make a decision in this area. However, it was vital in this case that the lady's close links with her father continued as this was of clear importance to them both.

3.6 Capacity assessment: Joint assessment – Inheritance

Background

A gentleman with a mild learning difficulty was referred to SLT by his GP to provide advice on how to support him in making his own decisions. The gentleman had recently inherited a significant sum of money from his aunt. Social services had raised concerns over the gentleman's ability to manage the finances now available to him and to identify whether he required a deputy to manage his financial affairs.

Action

The gentleman met with the SLT and GP, with whom he had a good relationship, at his GP's surgery. The professionals involved took into account advice from the MCA Code of Practice (2007) on how the gentleman should be helped to make his own decisions, such as:

• Providing relevant information

• Communicating in an appropriate way

• Making the person feel at ease

• Consideration of how someone can be helped to make a decision,

The session at the GP surgery established the level of the gentleman's understanding in relation to the source of his inheritance and the associated potential risks and benefits of receiving a large amount of money.

Outcome

After the session, the gentleman worked on developing a list of what he might like to spend his money on. This included items such as a new television and also smaller day-to-day treats as part of his food shopping. He was able to identify some risks of having an increase in wealth, for example people taking advantage of him and his money. He showed an ability to manage this; asserting his opinion about what he was happy spending his money on, for example, "I would like to buy a football ticket for me and my friend as I like to have someone to go to football with but I wouldn't treat him to more than that". It was agreed that this gentleman did have capacity to manage his finances.

3.7 Capacity versus compliance: Medical treatment

The MCA often covers decisions related to receiving healthcare. However, there are situations in which consideration needs to be given to the possible consequences of decision making and sometimes issues which initially appear to be related to capacity to consent need to be given further consideration. One such case is considered below.

Background

A gentleman was initially referred to SLT for an assessment of his capacity to consent to issues related to his ongoing health needs. The gentleman referred was in his 30s with mental health issues, a forensic history and a mild learning disability. He had been an inpatient in a secure hospital for three years and had recently been discharged back into the community to live with his wife.

The gentleman had kidney failure and consequently his hospital consultant had advised he begin dialysis. The gentleman was recommended to attend a local dialysis clinic three times every week for at least four hours each time. Dialysis is an artificial way of carrying out the process of cleaning and removing waste products from the body. This is usually carried out by the kidneys. Dialysis diverts the circulatory system through a dialysis machine in this process. Unfortunately, a kidney transplant was not an option for this gentleman.

The gentleman was not always compliant with dialysis and often did not attend appointments for several weeks, refusing to answer the door or becoming aggressive to staff when he did attend. At the point of non-compliance, staff became concerned about his capacity to consent to treatment.

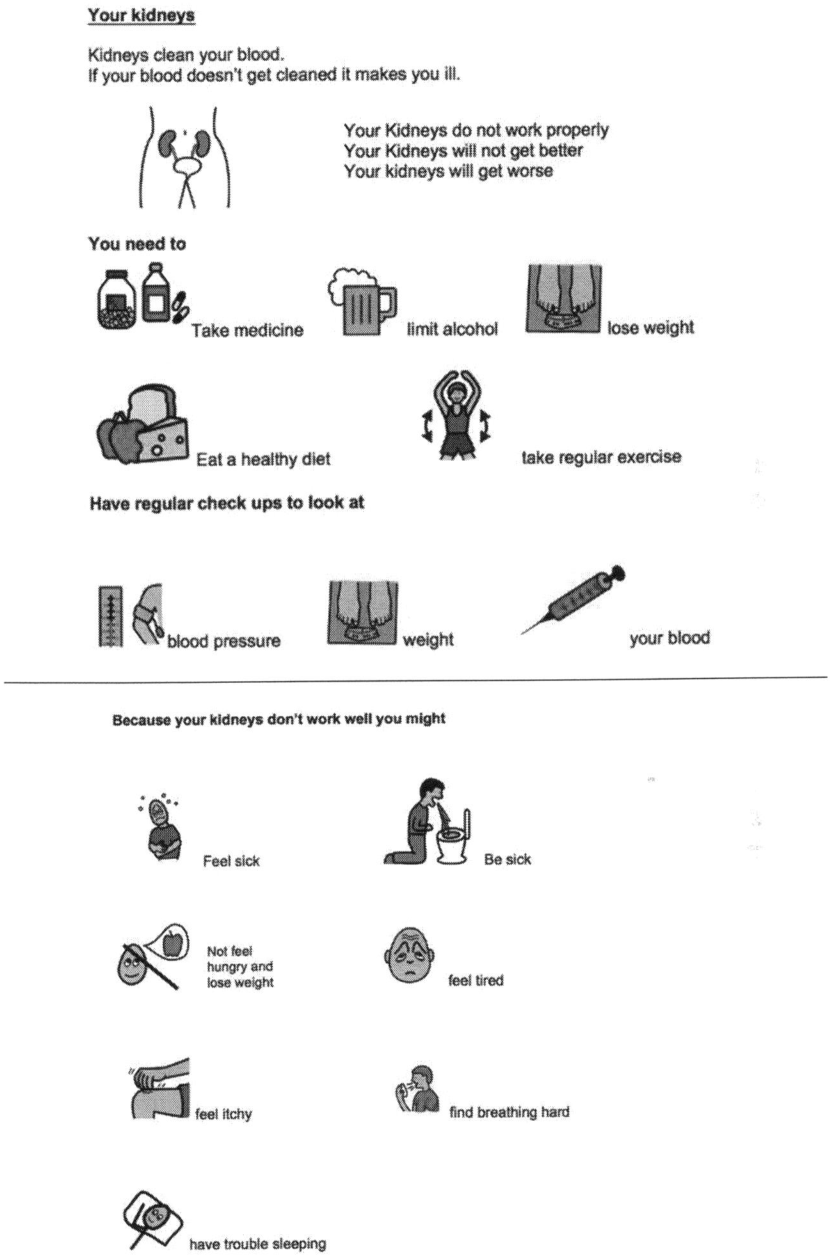

Your kidneys

Kidneys clean your blood.
If your blood doesn't get cleaned it makes you ill.

Your Kidneys do not work properly
Your Kidneys will not get better
Your kidneys will get worse

You need to

Take medicine   limit alcohol   lose weight

Eat a healthy diet   take regular exercise

Have regular check ups to look at

blood pressure   weight   your blood

Because your kidneys don't work well you might

Feel sick   Be sick

Not feel
hungry and
lose weight   feel tired

feel itchy   find breathing hard

have trouble sleeping

Figure 2.6 Example resources to support discussions.

Action

On meeting with the hospital consultant as decision maker in this case a discussion was held regarding the information related to the MCA. As this gentleman was not complying with health treatment, which had life-limiting implications it was questioned whether he had capacity to consent. During a discussion around this issue the team agreed that if the gentleman was not compliant with dialysis, then it would not be possible to complete dialysis. Thus, in this case the issue was identified as compliance and not capacity.

Outcome

In this circumstance, the role of SLT was to educate the gentleman in dialysis and kidney management (see some of the resources used in Figure 2.6). Additional work took place with other professionals such as the psychologist, to work through psychological issues which affected the gentleman's compliance and areas related to his treatment that he could control. This gentleman continues to attend dialysis inconsistently and manages his health on his own terms.

3.8 Capacity assessment: Facilitator – Medical procedure (Sexually Transmitted Infection – STI screening)

Background

A woman was referred to the SLT to facilitate a capacity to consent assessment in regard to a decision to have an internal examination to screen for sexually transmitted infections (STI). She was in her 20s, with a moderate learning disability and autism. She lived in a residential home and had 24-hour support from staff. The service user's psychologist agreed to be the decision maker in this area and the SLT's role was to facilitate communication during the assessment.

Action

The SLT phoned the sexual health clinic where the service user would have the screening to establish the step-by-step process that would occur. The SLT then produced accessible information for the service user regarding the nature of a STI, the consequence of having a STI and the screening process. This was made accessible after a baseline communication assessment had taken place to assess her level of understanding. The SLT gave the service user the opportunity to understand the accessible information over three separate visits. The SLT asked the service user questions throughout to informally assess her understanding of the information. The service user's comprehension and retention of the information increased noticeably over the three visits.

The psychologist and SLT then met with the woman and carried out the capacity to consent assessment involving:

1. Understanding the information relevant to the decision; such as, in her case, what a STI was, how a STI was transmitted, the consequences of having a STI, the process of screening for a STI. Questions were asked such as, "Where do you find bad sex germs?" and "How do you get bad sex germs?" ('bad sex germs' was used rather than 'sexually transmitted infection' as this was considered more accessible for the service user), "What will the nurse do?" to assess her understanding of the process of STI screening.

2. Retaining the information relevant to the decision. "What have I come to talk about?" was asked at the beginning of the session to assess whether the service user could retain information from the SLT's last visit. *(NB: retention is not required between session only for time required to make the decision.)*

3. Using or weighing up the information relevant to the decision; such as, in her case, what could be the good things about having a STI screen/STI, what could be the bad things about having a STI screen/STI.

4. Communicating her decision.

Outcome

The assessment demonstrated that with accessible information the service user was able to understand the information, retain it, weigh it up and express her decision to have STI screening. It was agreed that the service user had capacity to consent to this specific decision.

References

Adults with Incapacity (Scotland) Act Code of Practice (3rd edition, 2010). www.gov.scot/ Resource/Doc/327864/0105906.pdf

Aldous, K., Tolmie, R., Worrall, L., & Ferguson, A. (2014). Speech-Language Pathologists' contributions to the assessment of decision-making capacity in aphasia: A survey of common practices. *International Journal of Speech-Language Pathology, 16*(3), 231–241.

Belbin, R.M. (2010). *Team Roles at Work*, 2nd ed. London: Butterworth Heinemann.

Berne, E. (1961). *Transactional Analysis in Psychotherapy*. New York: Grove Press, Inc.

Carling-Rowland, A., Black, S., McDonald, L., & Kagan, A. (2014) Increasing access to fair capacity evaluation for discharge decision-making for people with aphasia: A randomized controlled trial. *Aphasiology, 28*(6), 750–765.

Cook, D.A., Brydges, R., Zendejas, B., Hamstra, S.J., & Hatala, R. (2013). Mastery learning for health professionals using technology-enhanced simulation: A systematic review and meta-analysis. *Academic Medicine, 88*(8), 1178-1186.

Devereux, C., Jackson, J., Marjoribanks, J., Harris, C., & Volkmer, A. (2016). Let's talk about capacity. *RCSLT Bulletin, 771*, 12-14.

Health Education England and Skills for Care (2015). Dementia Core Skills Education and Training Framework. Skills for Health.

Ferguson, A., Duffield, G., & Worrall, L. (2010). Legal decision-making by people with aphasia: Critical incidents for speech pathologists. *International Journal of Language and Communication Disorders, 45*(2), 244–268.

Forsgren, E., Hartelius, L., & Saldert, C. (2017). Improving medical students' knowledge and skill in communicating with people with acquired communication disorders. *International Journal of Speech-Language Pathology, 19*(6), 541–550.

Frenk, J., Chen, L., Bhutta, Z.A., Cohen, J., Crisp, N., Evans, T., ... & Kistnasamy, B. (2010). Health professionals for a new century: Transforming education to strengthen health systems in an interdependent world. *The Lancet, 376*(9756), 1923–1958.

General Medical Council (2013). Good Medical Practice. http://www.gmc-uk.org/guidance/ ethical_guidance/consent_guidance_accessing_capacity.asp

Hauer, P., Straub, C., & Wolf, S. (2005). Learning styles of allied health students using Kolb's LSI-IIa. *Journal of Allied Health, 34*(3), 177–182.

House of Lords (2014). Mental Capacity Act 2005: Post-legislative scrutiny. http://www. parliament.uk/mental- capacity-act-2005/

Karpman, S. (1968). Fairy tales and script drama analysis. *Transactional Analysis Bulletin, 7*(26), 39–43.

Knab, M., Inzana, R.S., Cahn, P.S., & Reidy, P.A. (2017, November). Preparing future health professionals for interprofessional collaborative practice. Part 2: The student experience. In *Seminars in Speech and Language*, Vol. 38, No. 05, pp.342-349. Thieme Medical Publishers.

Kolb, D.A. (1984). *Experiential Learning: Experience as the Source of Learning and Development*, Vol. 1. Englewood Cliffs, NJ: Prentice-Hall.

Laschinger, H.K. & Boss, M.W. (1984). Learning styles of nursing students and career choices. *Journal of Advanced Nursing, 9*(4), 375–380.

Luff, H. & Volkmer, A. (2016). Roles and relationships in the multidisciplinary team when assessing mental capacity In A. Volkmer (2016), *Dealing with Capacity and Other Legal Issues with Adults with Acquired Neurological Conditions: A Guide for SLTs.* Guildford: J&R Press.

Manee, F., Nadar, M., & Jahrami, H. (2013). Learning styles of allied health sciences students at Kuwait University. *International Journal of Therapy and Rehabilitation, 20*(5), 255–259.

McCarthy, J.W. & DiGiovanni, J.J. (2017, November). The interprofessional education environment: Places and pedagogies. In *Seminars in Speech and Language*, Vol. 38, No. 05, pp.368–380. Thieme Medical Publishers.

McCormick, M., Bose, A., & Marinis, T. (2017). Decision-making capacity in aphasia: SLT's contribution in England. *Aphasiology, 31*(11), 1344–1358.

Mental Capacity Act 2005: http://www.legislation.gov.uk/ukpga/2005/9/pdfs/ukpga_20050009_en.pdf

Mental Capacity Act 2005 Code of Practice (2007): http://www.legislation.gov.uk/ukpga/2005/9/pdfs/ukpgacop_20050009_en.pdf

O'Brien, R., Goldberg, S. E., Pilnick, A., Beeke, S., Schneider, J., Sartain, K., ... & Harwood, R. H. (2018). The VOICE study–A before and after study of a dementia communication skills training course. *PloS one, 13*(6), e0198567.

Saldert, C., Forsgren, E., & Hartelius, L. (2016). Teaching medical students about communication in speech-language disorders: Effects of a lecture and a workshop .*International Journal of Speech-Language Pathology, 18*(6), 571–579.

Royal College of Speech and Language Therapy (RCSLT) (2014). Submission from the Royal College of Speech and Language Therapists to the Department of Health, Social Services and Public Safety and the Department of Justice's Consultation on proposals for the Draft Mental Capacity Bill, Northern Ireland. http://www.rcslt.org/governments/docs/draft_mentalcapacity_bill

Royal College of Speech and Language Therapy (RCSLT) (2017). *Mental Capacity Factsheet.* https://www.rcslt.org/speech_and_language_therapy/slts_factsheets

Royal College of Speech and Language Therapy (RCSLT) (2014). Position Paper: *Speech and Language Therapy in Adult Critical Care.* http://www.rcslt.org/members/publications/publications2/criticalcare_positionpaper_060114

Royal College of Speech and Language Therapy (RCSLT) (2014). Position Paper: *SLT Provision for People with Dementia.* http://www.rcslt.org/members/publications/publications2/dementia_position_paper2014

Suleman, S. & Hopper, T. (2016). Decision-making capacity and aphasia: Speech-language pathologists' perspectives. *Aphasiology, 30*(4), 381–395.

Volkmer, A. (2016). *Dealing with Capacity and Other Legal Issues with Adults with Acquired Neurological Conditions: A Guide for SLTs.* Guildford: J&R Press.

Volkmer, A., Spector, A., Warren, J.D. & Beeke, S. (2018) Speech and Language Therapy for Primary Progressive Aphasia: Referral patterns and barriers to service provision across the UK. Dementia https://doi.org/10.1177/1471301218797240.

Wu, W., Martin, B.C., & Ni, C. (2017). A systematic review of competency-based education effort in the health professions: Seeking order out of chaos. *Handbook on Research on Competency-based Education in University Settings,* 352–378.

Zoghi, M., Brown, T., Williams, B., Roller, L., Jaberzadeh, S., Palermo, C., ... & Hewitt, L. (2010). Learning style preferences of Australian health science students. *Journal of Allied Health, 39*(2), 95–103.

Zuscak, S.J., Peisah, C., & Ferguson, A. (2016). A collaborative approach to supporting communication in the assessment of decision-making capacity. *Disability and Rehabilitation, 38*(11), 1107–1114.

3 Training teams to understand and implement the Mental Capacity Act (2005)

James Godber

Introduction

Speech and language therapists (SLTs) are uniquely placed to participate in mental capacity assessments. This is because SLTs have a detailed understanding of how communication of verbal and nonverbal information occurs. They have daily insights into what happens when communication of information breaks down and how best to support and repair interactions when breakdowns occur. This ability to recognize how to shape and manipulate the component parts of communicative interactions allows SLTs to support the optimal transfer of information between clinicians, service users and carers. SLTs can and do work with multiple stakeholders on facilitating access to the 'key' information in an interaction. These skills are vital for many capacity assessments; indeed, the Mental Capacity Act Code of Practice (2007) and the General Medical Council (2013) recommend seeking the professional opinion an SLT to support capacity assessments when individuals have complex communication difficulties.

SLTs are also well placed to use their expertise and experience to provide training to others in how to support individuals with communication difficulties in issues surrounding decision making and mental capacity. Communication skills training is addressed in detail in Chapter 5 of this book.

This chapter focuses on training teams to understand and implement the Mental Capacity Act (MCA, 2005) itself. It describes an approach to training a wide variety of healthcare professionals, including SLTs in understanding and using key parts of the legislation in their working lives. It is based on the experiences of the author, who has worked in both speech and language therapy services and safeguarding teams in a hospital setting. The training described highlights the enabling ethos of the MCA and describes a supportive approach to decision making. Detailed scenarios, training content, and discussion starters are included.

The case studies presented later in this chapter highlight the benefit of a collaborative approach to practice when it comes to applying the MCA. For complex and serious decisions, joint working, clear communication and shared reasoning are particularly essential. Given this, it is perhaps unsurprising that feedback on training we have provided locally has indicated that when training is attended by a range of multidisciplinary team professionals it is more effective. It has also emphasized that attendees value interactive training and case studies which enable trainees to practice applying the key elements of the Act. Some published research also supports interactive training, describing using discursive, scenario based examples to help practitioners understand relevant theory and legislation (see Gough & Kerlin, 2012; Marshall & Sprung, 2016; Wilson,Seymour, & Perkins, 2010).

The training proposed in this chapter describes six suggested stages for a thorough, interactive training session:

1. Finding out what people think the MCA is about.

2. Exploring how trainees make their own decisions.

3. Exploring and highlighting reasons for ineffective implementation of the MCA.

4. Explaining obligations under the MCA and the implications of ignoring or diluting them.

5. Practical tips on training health professionals to support decision making and assess capacity in line with the MCA.

6. Working together and managing conflict: Navigating a consensus approach to implementing the MCA.

1 Finding out what people think the MCA is about

To achieve participant engagement the trainer must establish what the participants know of the MCA and also convince the trainees of the relevance of the MCA and the training to their jobs and lives. Understanding of the

MCA may be highly variable. Finding out what 'capacity' means to trainees, and their thoughts on using the Act in their clinical roles, can be a useful starting point. Early exploration of how we make decisions for ourselves can help trainees relate legislation to freedom of choice in their own lives; this is discussed at more length in Section II of this chapter.

The demand for 'bite-size' learning in busy and resource-limited healthcare settings is a challenge irrespective of the subject being discussed. Training focused on 'concrete' areas such as manual handling, hand hygiene, and resuscitation provides people with a mental picture of what to expect from a session before they enter the training room. In comparison, mental capacity may be a much more abstract concept to many. This can be a challenge when considering how to practically apply capacity-related legislation to daily practice. Clinicians may have had minimal exposure to training on capacity (Marshall & Sprung, 2016). It can be helpful to discuss and acknowledge this at the beginning of a session, with the aim of putting people who feel less confident about the Act at ease. Acknowledging the national picture with regards to the MCA can be useful. As the 2014 House of Lords Select Committee report on the MCA outlines:

> "The Act has suffered from a lack of awareness and a lack of understanding. For many who are expected to comply with the Act it appears to be an optional add-on, far from being central to their working lives." (p.8)

Even healthcare professionals who have had training, and may have an intellectual awareness of the MCA and its relevance to clinical practice, may have difficulty, or feel less confident, in actually applying it to their day-to-day working life (Gough & Kerlin, 2012; Wilson et al., 2010). As overall practice relating to the MCA is probably best described as variable (see HM Government NMCF Annual Report 2016 for a summary), establishing a degree of baseline knowledge via informal discussion can help appropriately focus a training session.

Knowing the settings where participants work can also be useful, allowing a focus on relevant clinical scenarios during the session. These scenarios should focus on clinical interactions with service users. Example questions that may encourage initial discussion and enable a better understanding of the knowledge and experience of attendees are summarized in Table 3.1.

Table 3.1 Suggested questions for eliciting discussion around the understanding of the MCA and how it is applied to practice.

What do you know about the MCA?
When do you use the MCA?
Can you think of examples of care and treatment options and decisions that a service user you're working with might face?
What conditions do you associate with a difficulty in thinking or communicating?
Can you think of people you have worked with who have had difficulty thinking or communicating? How did you manage this?
Can you think of an example of when you have been worried about a service user's capacity to make a decision?
How do you manage situations when someone refused care of treatment that you really think they need?
What does best interests mean to you?
What is the role of family member/clinician when a service user does not have the capacity to decide on a course of action themselves?

Defining the Act simply, in a way that relates to communicative interactions

Responses to questions set out in Table 3.1 will elicit discussion that can be supplemented with an accessible overview of the ethos of the Act. The Social Care Institute of Excellence's website (https://www.scie.org.uk) provides a useful summary, outlining the Act as:

> "designed to protect and restore power to those vulnerable people who may lack capacity to make certain decisions, due to the way their mind is affected by illness or disability, or the effects of drugs or alcohol".

Highlighting the idea of restoring or optimizing a person's ability to communicate *their own* decisions can be valuable. When correctly applied, the MCA minimizes the chances of decisions being made arbitrarily on behalf of someone else. Put simply, the MCA is 'about making decisions'. The four key questions, set out in Table 3.2, provide a practical tool to highlight how the Principles of the MCA can be applied.

Table **3.2** Four-step summary to using the MCA to support care and treatment decisions.

1. Have I provided the key relevant information to the service user about a care and treatment intervention/option and checked that they understand?

2. Do I have a reason to think that this person has a difficulty with thinking or communication that may be affecting their ability to make full use this information?

3. If yes, how can this person be best and most neutrally supported to access and convey information that allows them to share their own individual decision?

4. If all reasonable efforts to support this person to make their own individual decision fail, how can I still support them with the aim of their will and preferences having the maximum possible impact on any decision made for them?

Highlighting the enabling aspects of the MCA

Explaining the MCA as a continuum of support that enables people to be involved is useful. Our approach should always start with the aim of enabling people to retain maximum control over care and treatment decisions (see Figure 3.1). As SLTs we can be on comfortable ground with the idea of the supportive approach shown in Figure 3.1. Training others to consider this supportive

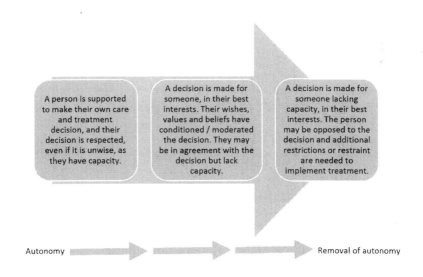

Autonomy ▷▷▷ ▷▷▷ ▷▷▷ Removal of autonomy

Figure 3.1 Continuum of enabling decision making.

approach can start with the idea of shelving "all thoughts of a capacity assessment and providing 'all practicable steps to support the person to make the decision'" (Currie, 2016, from presentation).

It is worth emphasizing that taking this approach means anticipating all the steps required to make the decision in question and preparing appropriately so that individuals receive the support they need. This would typically involve: a full assessment; gathering a history; speaking with the necessary individuals; and gathering people and resources together as appropriate to support the person.

Although a supportive approach is required by law, it is often missing in practice and documentation. Referrals made to the safeguarding team often relate to the 'end' of the MCA continuum, including cases where Deprivations of Liberty Safeguards (DoLs) are being considered. By this stage, a working relationship with the service user has often broken down, and it may seem that the professionals involved are requesting the safeguarding team to legitimize a decision taken to keep a person where they are against their wishes. For example, the timing of such referrals may coincide with increased difficulty managing an individual's behaviour, a desire to prevent them leaving the hospital because of concerns about their safety, and perhaps even frustration at a perceived inability of an individual to 'be reasonable' and prioritize the clinical elements of a decision facing them. This can lead to broad statements in medical notes, such as 'patient clearly lacks capacity' or 'patient confused so procedure undertaken in best interests'. Forensic investigation of the lead-up to such DoL requests can sometimes reveal shortening or omitting of aspects of the MCA, that should precede a 'best interest decision' (and the use of any restrictions used to 'keep them safe'). The evidence of support, that might have enabled an individual to stay in control of their own choices, may be lacking. Additionally, the non-clinical factors that might have contributed to their decision may remain hidden (due to conversations left uninitiated and questions unasked). This is clearly an area for development and well worth dedicating some time to during a training session.

2 Exploring how trainees make their own decisions

At the start of a training session it can be helpful to ask trainees to think about how they arrive at everyday versus more serious decisions. Even everyday questions such as "how did you decide what to have for breakfast this morning?" can reveal the structured approach people routinely and quickly apply to decision making. Currie (2016) suggests using an example such as "I would like to offer you a new job, are you going to accept?" to elicit the kind of strategies people would undertake in order to make a more important or substantial decision.

Typical responses from training participants about what they would do if offered the 'mystery' job include statements such as "I'd need to understand what the job is [pay, location, area of work, skillset]", "I'd need to ask questions", "I'd need time to think", "I'd need to know if it fits in with my life", "I'd want to talk it through with family", "I'd want to talk to someone working in that field to find out more", "I'd make a list of pros and cons", "I'd pray/sleep on it". Currie also outlines that decision making is not always perfect on the first attempt and is not always based on cold, robotic logic but is personal and subjective. Most people in training sessions seem able to relate to the idea that you might have an immediate reaction to a decision that you later return to and change following the benefits of measured reflection. Or that you might have almost made up your mind but are then swayed by the opinion of someone you trust. Or that you might not be sure what to do and prefer to leave it to fate, or the flip of a coin.

Asking the participants to reflect on decision making in their own lives can raise insight into the needs of people *without* communication and with cognitive difficulties. This may include the need to clearly understand what the decision is, the ability to explore options and alternatives, gather information and have the time, resources and support of others to do so, in a way that works for them. This may help people move away from a more superficial approach to supporting more vulnerable service users with communication and cognitive difficulties to make decisions. In other words, going beyond hearing aids, glasses and a few communication aids to survive a capacity assessment (important though these might be) and a movement away from capacity assessment feeling like a test or exam.

Having reflected on their own decision-making processes the next stage of training can focus on more relevant issues. For example, the following questions could be discussed:

- How much of the language used in healthcare settings is technical, or likely to require explanation to someone who is not a healthcare professional?

- How much time and support do you think a cognitively intact service user with no communication difficulties typically has when they need to make a decision about their health care?

- How many times have you had a follow-up conversation with such a service user about a treatment or procedure that has been 'explained' to them, only to find that they had taken away inaccurate or insufficient information about that treatment?

Questions like this may also highlight the potential power imbalance that exists when a service user who may have impaired capacity enters a healthcare provider's domain (NMCF Annual Report, HM Government, 2016). Before implementation of the MCA is at all necessary it is important to try and create an environment where all service users believe the decision is theirs to make. Irrespective of communication or cognitive impairments, people may lack confidence in decision making, they may be ill, in shock, confused, scared or not used to making decisions for themselves (Joshi, 2015). None of these factors necessarily mean they are incapacitated, but they may indicate that thoughtful and considered support is required. The level of support required is likely to be greater if someone has an impairment of, or disturbance in, the functioning of their mind or brain.

Highlighting decision making conversations that occur regularly in practice

Having discussed the drivers behind decision making and their importance to participants in general, it can then be helpful to explore common interactions or clinical scenarios where healthcare decision making takes place. Depending on the professional background of people attending training, a profession-specific approach may be useful here (see Chapter 6 of Volkmer, 2016, for a review of the potential roles of different multidisciplinary team (MDT) professionals in relation to mental capacity). Where trainees come from a mixture of different professional backgrounds, a small portfolio of scenarios that a range of healthcare professionals can relate to may be most useful. Table 3.3 provides a non-exhaustive list of some of these scenarios.

Discussion using case scenarios can be a really useful part of a training session. Trainees often share attitudes, approaches and areas of good and bad practice that they or others have experienced. Working with trainees to reflect these cases can also focus on: how the information is being presented; linking practice to the principles of the MCA; reflecting on any gaps between the delivery and content of less optimal conversations; and comparing accessible, neutral and unbiased approaches to meet the requirements of the MCA.

Table 3.3 Flashpoints: Common interactions in healthcare settings where explanations, discussions and decision making can occur.

Routine care interventions, e.g., supporting turning and personal hygiene.

Administration of medications. Insertion/removal of lines/tubes associated with treatment.

Discussion and provision of routine medical and therapy interventions.

Considering, applying or replacing restrictions, e.g., bed rails, mittens, pharmacological restraint, introduction or maintenance of 1:1 supervision. Restricting service user's freedom of movement within a particular location.

Conversations with service users who wish to self-discharge against medical or clinical advice.

Conversations with service users about serious medical or surgical treatment decisions.

Non-oral feeding/risk feeding decisions.

Discharge planning including where a change of accommodation is being considered.

Table 3.4 Feedback from participants on interactions with service users relating to care and treatment decisions.

"They were pretty agitated and confused, and refused to be turned even though I told them they had a pressure sore. I was worried about it getting worse but I let them be. I'm not going to force someone." (Member of the nursing team)

"I went to talk to a service user after the speech therapist had seen them. The speech therapist had put them nil by mouth but they were asking me to give them a drink. I know the speech therapist had tried to explain to them but they were surprised when I told them they couldn't have a drink and got quite angry with me." (HCA)

"Everyone knows consent is a bit of a joke really. As the professional, you know how to ask questions in a way that gets the answers that fit with your clinical recommendations – which you arrive at with the service user's best interests at heart." (Doctor)

"They said, you know, with all these falls, it's going to be better for you to live somewhere where you can get some proper care. You don't want to come back into hospital any time soon do you? The service user, of course, said, "no, definitely not." (AHP feedback on a family meeting)

"So we spent a week working with the service user to understand and remember the risks. I was really surprised at how their insight developed. It really improved our relationship too, as before they'd just refused the idea of care and just wanted to leave but in the end they agreed to it and think they really understood why it was needed." (Doctor)

"I just wanted to thank you for allowing me to make my own decision on this. I know it's taken me a long time to do it, and I knew that what you were recommending was the right thing, but I had to get there myself." (Service user)

Some people often raise issues at this point that hint at the underlying personal and institutional barriers that may obstruct implementation of the MCA. These may include having inadequate time, a desire to persuade people to take the least possible risk, and feeling uncomfortable discussing concerns with colleagues. Other trainees may provide valuable insights into positive outcomes that occur when enabling steps are worked into interactions from the offset. Some anonymized examples of feedback are detailed in Table 3.4.

3 Exploring and highlighting reasons for ineffective implementation of the MCA

Much of the local feedback from trainees relating to decision making 'flashpoints' will reflect findings from national work investigating difficulties in implementing the MCA. Being aware of these findings can help the trainer anticipate the barriers trainees may face. Additionally, summarizing key themes during the training may help people recognize and perhaps avoid some of these. The following six issues are particularly useful to consider.

1 Reduced knowledge and awareness of the Act itself and/or reduced systems and processes to support routine application

Several studies identify insufficient training for staff in understanding and applying the MCA (see Marshall & Sprung, 2016, for an overview and further references). There is also evidence that awareness of the Act and knowledge and confidence in relation to the MCA can be poor (Gough & Kerlin, 2012; Herring, 2009; Marshall & Sprung, 2016; Wilner et al., 2013) even amongst senior and specialist clinicians.

In the hierarchical world of healthcare, reduced knowledge at a senior level may adversely affect the promotion of a consultative, interdisciplinary, consensus-based approach in relation to the MCA. There is also the possibility, in this environment, that senior staff may react defensively if challenged (Phair & Manthorpe, 2012). If application of the MCA is not well understood at an organizational level, then this may reduce the chances of it being integrated into clinical systems, discussions, routines and paperwork.

It can be valuable to acknowledge these as common difficulties that have been experienced across the country (House of Lords, 2014; HM Government, 2016). Learning how to implement the MCA should be seen as a process that takes time. This may help take the pressure off trainees to know everything they need to after a 60-minute session, free them up to ask 'stupid' questions, and encourage them to seek support and work with others when implementing the MCA. Encouraging teams to embed the MCA into their systems (discussions, routines and paperwork) in the form of reminders or prompts can be a realistic and useful strategy.

2 Inconsistent application of the two-stage test/misunderstanding of Principle 1

Misunderstanding or misuse of Principle 1 is a well-documented issue. The presumption of capacity (i.e., every adult has the right to make his or her own decisions unless there is evidence to the contrary) can be misinterpreted in two key ways. Firstly, some people, secondary to a condition they have, or a behaviour they exhibit "may be expected to prove that they have capacity for a decision, rather than capacity being assumed until proved otherwise" (NMCF Annual Report, HM Government, 2016, p. 28). This can lead to discrimination against people who may have been able to make those decisions themselves (this not uncommon for people with aphasia). Conversely, if capacity is assumed when there is reason to suspect that an impairment of a person's brain or mind is impacting upon their ability to make a particular decision, then a vulnerable person who lacks decision-making capacity may be exposed to adverse consequences of the decision outcome, unforeseen by themselves. This is not an uncommon experience for some individuals with traumatic brain injury. These individuals may be assumed to have capacity to make a decision when in fact their reduced insight and awareness as a result of their brain injury mean they are unable to appreciate the consequence of their decision on their own lives.

As the House of Lords Select Committee report (2014, Chapter 3, p. 105) outlines: "The presumption of capacity, in particular, is widely misunderstood by those involved in care. It is sometimes used to support non-intervention or poor care, leaving vulnerable adults exposed to risk of harm. This may be because professionals struggle to understand how to apply the principle in practice (although a more deliberate 'misuse' of Principle 1 of the MCA has been cited in some cases to deliberately avoid taking responsibility for a vulnerable adult)".

Table 3.5 provides an example conversation with follow-up questions to explore presumption of capacity. It is always interesting to find that, whilst most participants are able to identify that the decision is around deciding to eat and drink by mouth there are always a number of participants who answer 'yes' to the second question. Follow-up discussions with people who have said 'yes' suggest they were strongly influenced by the way Peter was unambiguously able to communicate what he wanted and some refer to the Principle 1 as the reason for arriving at their decision, e.g., "Well, yes, I think he has capacity, I mean like you said, I think we have to presume capacity,

Table 3.5 Example conversation.

Background: Peter in an 88-year-old man who has recently been admitted following a stroke. His swallow has been assessed by speech and language therapy and, as Peter appears to be at high risk of aspiration on oral intake, he has been placed NBM and an NG tube has been placed. It is lunchtime and other service users' meals are arriving.
Peter: Nurse.
HCA: Yes, Peter.
Peter: Can I have some lunch.
HCA: No, the speech therapist has seen you. Your swallow isn't working.
Peter: I'm swallowing fine. I've never had a problem swallowing.
HCA: Sorry, Peter, It's not safe.
Peter: This is ridiculous, you're trying to starve me. I want to eat something now and I'm very thirsty. Please get me some food and drink.
Question 1: What is the decision?
Question 2: Does Peter have capacity to make this decision?

and he's clearly communicating that he wants to eat and drink". Those who responded 'no' often cite the stroke as a reason to doubt his capacity, or the notion that he has not taken on board the risks of taking food and drink by mouth, indicating a lack of capacity.

Analysis of simple exchanges such as this example conversation allows Principle 1 to be more fully explored. Further discussion can illustrate how the key guidance within the MCA relies on balanced use of the different parts of the act. This discussion may include:

• The presumption of capacity shouldn't be overruled just because an impairment of mind or brain is present (in Peter's case, the underlying condition in question is a stroke). He may well have capacity to make such a decision irrespective of his stroke.

• Whilst we might make assumptions (for example that Peter has had an explanation from the SLT and that he has or has not processed it), we can't effectively consider this issue based solely on the basis of this interaction. This is because, in this interaction, Peter hasn't been provided with enough support to understand the key reasons why it might be 'unsafe' for him to swallow (Principle 2 of the MCA) and the subsequent opportunity to demonstrate, perhaps via such a conversation, whether or not he can understand, recall and weigh that key information to arrive at a decision, that may be unwise (in line with Principle 3).

- The answer to the question of whether or not Peter has capacity should be: "I don't know. Further conversation or more support is required to answer that question."

3 Behavioural or professional/institutional resistance to the principles of the Act

Healthcare professionals requesting support in cases where capacity has been questioned are sometimes motivated in part by a desire to steer the service user away from a potentially unwise decision to the safest course of action relating to a decision. This risk reduction approach is understandable in an increasingly litigious society but arguably it also reflects the paternalism that remains prevalent in many healthcare settings. As the House of Lords Report (2014, Chapter 1, 14) summarizes:

> "A consistent theme in the evidence was the tension between the empowerment which the Act was designed to deliver, and the tendency of professionals to use the Act for safeguarding purposes. Prevailing professional cultures of risk aversion and paternalism have inhibited the aspiration of empowerment from being realised".

It can be valuable to explore this point in training by acknowledging that protecting someone from a decision that might be considered unreasonable or unsafe is entirely understandable and fits well with the maxim of 'do no harm'. It may, though, conflict with the MCA's ethos of giving equal credence to an individual's right to make unwise decisions (if they have capacity) that are right for them, even if such a decision might directly lead to a worse physical outcome for that person, including their death (EWCOP 80, [2015] MHLO 125).

However, whether motivated by benevolent paternalism, a fear of litigation, or their own values and beliefs, healthcare professionals may view unwise decisions negatively (Atwal, McIntyre, & Wiggett, 2011; Lamont, Jeon, & Chiarella, 2013). Regarding personal bias, it may help trainees to bear in mind that case law, even prior to the introduction of the MCA, included advice that clinicians "must not allow their emotional reaction to, or strong disagreement with, the decision of the service user to cloud their judgment in answering the primary question whether the service user has the mental capacity to make

Table 3.6 Examples of unwise decision outside a healthcare setting.

"Regularly running across a busy road to get to the station when running late for my train."
"Eating three crispy crème doughnuts in one sitting."
"Smoking."
"Free climbing" (rock climbing without ropes).
"Leaving the engine running in my car while I pop into a shop."
"Saying yes to a third drink on a Friday night."

the decision" ([2002[EWHC 429 (Fam)). Case law has also supported the idea that clinicians may, at times, set the bar for capacity too high to allow people to make informed but unwise decisions ([2011] EWCH 1704 (Fam). Clinicians have an obligation under the MCA to support decision making and not to expect that an individual should demonstrate comprehensive expertise in a subject area to demonstrate capacity. Rather, they should be able to process the information relating to the 'key issues'.

Active discussion of a service user's rights to make unwise decisions under the MCA can reveal a protective and paternalistic approach at times. Trainees often reflect on this issue differently when asked to consider their own right to make unwise decisions. Typically, trainees report that they experience negative reactions when told that they shouldn't do something that someone else considered to be unwise, or because they 'don't know enough'. Table 3.6 provides a list of anonymized unwise decisions people might make in daily life. It can be useful to share these in training to illustrate this point.

Pitfalls of personal or professional prejudices can be avoided by making use of the steps enshrined in the Principles of the MCA: making sure someone is adequately supported to make an informed decision, and if there is still doubt about capacity, taking a structured approach to differentiating between in-capacitous and unwise decisions. The MCA framework, used correctly, optimizes the chance of consistent assessment, reduced subjectivity, personal prejudice and bias (Marshall & Sprung, 2016).

4 Poor spoken and written communication in relation to decision making and capacity

Breakdown in communication is a common theme when difficulties arise around decision making (see Luff & Volkmer, Ch. 6 in Volkmer, 2016). A lack of proactive, joined-up practice when supporting complex decision making can be a particular issue. This can include confusion about who is the 'decision maker' or the person responsible for supporting decision making or carrying out the capacity assessment. There is often an apparent lack of consultation with family members and significant others to provide key background information that might be relevant to a decision. Information held by one part of the team may not be shared with another in a timely and effective way. Information sharing may be de-prioritized, or information may simply be ignored when it is shared. This can result in disagreements relating to whether or not a service user has capacity, and what action may be in their best interests. Requests for support in managing these issues may be delayed or not made, risking escalation of the issues at hand.

Disagreement between professionals can result in confusion and frustration between members of the MDT, service users, and their families. Different health professionals are likely to hold knowledge of different interactions with service users and their significant others, and have a range of different skills and knowledge relating to risk assessment, cognition, mental health and communication. It is perhaps unsurprising that effective MDT working has been identified as a key component of effective implementation of the MCA (BPS (PPB) 2006). The case study below provides an example of what happens when lines of communication are poor.

Case study 1

Janet, a 36-year-old woman, was admitted for treatment of a serious condition related to reversible organ failure.

Her medical history included a stroke, two years earlier, which initially affected mobility, thinking, swallowing and communication. In the months following her stroke she had made a significant recovery. Her ability to mobilize within the house she shared with family improved, she was able to take normal food and fluids by mouth again, and returned to managing several household activities and accessing the community. Whilst her communication had improved, she still had moderate-to-severe expressive aphasia and moderate receptive as a result of the stroke.

During the early stages of her current admission, she presented as acutely unwell, and remained in bed for several weeks before she stabilized medically. She was nil by mouth with a Naso gastric tube to maintain her nutrition and hydration. Once medically stabilized, decompensation of her pre-existing function was noted across mobility, swallowing and the ability to participate in activities of daily living. Occupational therapy and physiotherapy received referrals to work with Janet on mobility, transfers and activities of daily living. SLT were asked to provide input to support a return to oral intake. SLT also provided incidental information on her level of communicative function and provided general recommendations. No further communication input was provided or requested. Comments from other members of the team relating to communication suggested that Janet had good use of social phrases, seemed to understand the doctors when they came to discuss her treatment, and appeared to follow instructions well in therapy tasks.

As time progressed, Janet was due to be transferred to her local hospital when a bed became available. Janet's swallow had improved and she started a normal diet and normal fluids at the recommendation of the SLT. However, occupational therapy and physiotherapy assessment indicated that whilst some recovery was evident, her level of function was not yet adequate for her to safely manage at home. At this point, Janet started to indicate that she wanted to go home and members of her family were also keen for her to be discharged. A junior doctor assessed her capacity to make this decision. He documented that she lacked capacity to self-discharge but did not provide any details of the interaction. Two other members of the team also reported on Janet's decision-making capacity in relation to this decision in the medical notes; one entry described uncertainty about whether or not Janet had capacity to make the decision to self-discharge, and another recorded that Janet 'probably does have capacity'. Minimal details of the interactions themselves were recorded.

Shortly after this, Janet was referred to the safeguarding team as she was attempting to self-discharge, with support of her family. Meetings were held where it was agreed that Janet lacked the decision-making capacity to return home based on her inability to understand and weigh up risks of returning home. However, due to Janet's level of distress when remaining on the ward, it was decided that it was in her best interest to return home. Several different agencies were involved in supporting

Janet and her family after discharge. However, a formal complaint was later made by the family, in which they outlined poor communication as a substantial factor in the breakdown of the relationships between family members (including Janet) and staff.

A post-discharge case review was initiated in which the following additional facts came to light:

1. Janet was very worried about her partner coping alone with the care burden as another elderly family member lived with them who had complex needs.

2. Janet's partner had been informed by a member of the medical team three days before he arrived that Janet was 'medically fit for discharge'. Janet was also present when this conversation occurred.

3. Janet's partner had called a junior doctor two days before the day of her discharge, stating his intention to take Janet home. This was verbally handed over to another member of the MDT but not documented.

4. Janet's partner had asked to meet with the MDT on more than one occasion but received no response.

5. Therapies had not spoken directly to Janet's family about discharge concerns.

6. Occupational therapy and physiotherapy, against a background of competing clinical demands, had reduced the frequency of their sessions with Janet due to refusal and poor compliance as well as a potential plan for her to transfer to another hospital, thus removing the impetus to escalate discharge planning.

7. Most individual members of the MDT were aware that Janet was keen to go home and that opinions were mixed about her capacity, but no MDT discussion had taken place about this in person until the day of her discharge.

Reflection points based on the review of this case:

- The risks of discharge could have been more clearly defined and shared earlier with Janet, MDT and family.

- Rather than de-prioritizing Janet's therapy sessions because she was not engaging, a broader approach to input could have been adopted to try and understand why she was objecting, and what more could be done to engage her closer to her own terms.

- The MDT could have requested SLT input to support interactions that might have helped Janet to access the rationale and aims of other therapy input and to support communication during the sessions.

- More efforts could have been made to find out about Janet's social background so that this information could have been considered.

- Documentation of conversations with Janet and family members could have been more rigorous and accurate.

- More could have been done to explain the meaning and limitations inherent in the term 'medically fit for discharge'.

- The MDT could have requested SLT input to support discussions relating to discharge risks and any ensuing capacity assessment.

- Discussions with Janet around capacity could have been shared, planned and agreed by the MDT, and conducted in a consistent way.

- Following variable opinion relating to Janet's capacity to self-discharge, joint capacity assessment could have been conducted with external support.

- Documentation relating to Janet's ability to make decisions could have been better.

There were too few opportunities for face-to-face cross-disciplinary discussion of these issues in the ward in question.

5 Inadequate capacity assessments

Local audit of implementation of the MCA reveals that in many cases capacity assessments haven't been completed or have been completed to an insufficient degree. These parallel findings from the 2017 London Safeguarding Adults

Board review which also noted flawed use of the MCA in this regard. Clinicians documenting incomplete capacity assessments may include a reference to a service user's general state of confusion and a need to make 'decisions' in their best interest. Statements such as 'patient lacks capacity' or 'patient has capacity' may be written without any explanation of how this conclusion was reached. The pathway to a finding of capacity or incapacity may also be based on inaccurate interpretation of the MCA, e.g., "patient clearly lacks capacity as they cannot remember what I said to them yesterday", or, "patient has capacity to consent to the operation as they consistently say 'yes' when I asked them if they want to go ahead".

Typically, documentation involving suboptimal capacity assessments features one or more of the following:

- The disorder of mind or brain is not linked to evidence of difficulty making a time-specific decision.

- The specific decision is not identified and/or there are multiple decisions lumped together with blanket capacity/incapacity stated.

- The key information required to make a decision (against which capacity will be judged) is unclear or unbalanced.

- Capacity is not judged against the specific decision but used as a general term.

- The four stages of capacity assessment have not all been tested (understanding, recalling, weighing/evaluating and communicating).

- The contents of the service user's responses are absent or not clearly detailed.

- Assessment appears to have been administered quickly and unilaterally, without other professionals who might have offered supporting knowledge and skills, or even just a second opinion.

Reduced confidence in administering or documenting assessment may be a contributory factor to a poverty or absence of documentation relating to capacity assessment, as might confusion about who should lead the capacity assessment or make the final judgement call on whether a person has the capacity to make a particular decision at a given time. Additionally, as previously mentioned, the amount and complexity of information a person might be expected to process in order to make a decision may be calibrated to 'achieve' a finding of capacity or incapacity to enable the outcome desired or recommended by the clinician.

However, it is also important to be aware of certain groups, for example people with traumatic brain injuries, who may appear to demonstrate an ability to 'jump through the hoops' of a capacity assessment (e.g., clearly recalling and identifying the risks relating to their well-communicated choice in a particular situation) but who may also lack the ability to effectively judge risk secondary to their injury. Such a presentation may require a more in-depth assessment of weighing and evaluating information by observing behaviour and action over time as well as formal assessments of decision-making capacity (see Acquired Brain Injury and MCA Interest Group, 2014, for recommended further reading).

A capacity assessment that is well administered and documented supports service users to make their own decisions wise or unwise in the eyes of the assessor, and will demonstrate clearly which of the stages of a capacity assessment an individual is unable to complete if they are found not to have capacity to make a particular decision. It should also protect the clinician from liability for the consequences of that decision if their actions are guided by the outcome of a robust and unbiased assessment. Decisions that are reached via circumvention or omission of part or all of an assessment of capacity are inadequate and open to litigation.

6 Narrow interpretation and truncated application of the Best Interests Decision Making Process

When trainees are asked if they have heard the term 'best interests' in a healthcare setting, there is usually a collective nod. When asked what 'best interests' actually means there is often hesitancy before anyone responds. Thereafter, trainees often divide into two camps. Some typically relate the term 'best interests' to a person's medical needs or their physical safety. Feedback may include comments such as, "whatever is going to stop them getting worse", or, "whatever will keep them safe". Others, though, may lead with comments such as "it depends what's right for them", pointing to consideration of non-clinical issues as part of a best interests' process. Subsequent discussion with trainees typically results in an acknowledgement that someone's personal and social factors, their approach to life, and perhaps their feelings about risk are often overlooked or sidelined in best interests' decision making, secondary to medical or clinical factors.

The House of Lords Select Committee report on the MCA (2014, Conclusions and Recommendations, 2) criticized a more 'narrow' interpretation, stating that "Best interests' decision-making is often not undertaken in the way set out in the Act: the wishes, thoughts and feelings of [the service user] are not routinely prioritised. Instead, clinical judgments or resource-led decision making predominate". It is important for trainees to consider that clinical factors should not always be prioritized in best interests' decision making. Case law supports the idea that even when a decision may result in an individual dying sooner than they otherwise would, it might still be in their best interests to reject the clinical recommendation (Briggs vs Briggs [2016] EWCOP provides a recent piece of supporting case law outlining this argument under the MCA).

Trainees should ideally leave training sessions with an understanding that unless a clinician is dealing with an emergency situation, a holistic approach to best interests' decision making should prevail. Certainly, for serious medical treatment and discharge decisions, consultation with the service user who lacks decision-making capacity and discussion with those close to them (who are likely to know a great deal more than the treating clinician about the service user's values, beliefs and past decisions) should be considered part of any best interests' decision-making process. Additionally, and without labouring the point, best interests' discussions should only occur when all reasonable attempts to support the service user to make their own decision have been exhausted without success.

4 Explaining obligations under the MCA and the implications of ignoring or diluting them

It can be useful to point out to trainees that the consequences of poor practice in relation to the MCA extend beyond the inappropriate removal of many of an individual's fundamental rights. Outlining the legal expectations relating to the MCA should include an overview of how healthcare bodies are judged on the presence and quality of their work relating to capacity, as this may help focus a range of health professionals on the key aspects of their approach to both practice and documentation. This topic may also be helpful should you need additional evidence to persuade senior stakeholders or budget holders of the value of providing training relating to the MCA. Poor practice can result in poor ratings for the organization, consequent loss of reputation, statutory warning notices, or even prosecution. There is also the possibility of costly and time-consuming litigation.

The House of Lords Select Committee Report (2014, Conclusions and Recommendations, Recommendation 16) recommended that "the standards against which the CQC inspects should explicitly incorporate compliance with the Mental Capacity Act". As a consequence of this HM Government (2016) released a statement emphasizing that (Recommendation 5, p. 2) "The CQC has significantly raised the profile of the MCA in its inspection regime" and that "The MCA is now a 'Key Line of Inquiry' during CQC inspections". They also referred to improved training and understanding of the MCA amongst Care Quality Commission (CQC) staff themselves. In short, the message, which has been borne out in recent CQC inspections, is that organizational implementation of the MCA is under increased and more focused scrutiny. Several recent CQC reports explicitly mention poor practice in relation to the MCA, under the domains 'effective' and 'caring'. For examples of recent reports relating to Hospital Trusts see: https://www.cqc.org.uk/search/services/all?f%5B0%5D=im_field_inspection_rating%3A3928&f%5B1%5D=im_field_popular_services%3A3672

Referring healthcare professionals to the CQC guidance for National Health Service (NHS) providers (particularly the sections of 'consent to care and treatment' and 'involving people in decisions about their care') can provide an accessible overview of the indicators of good practice an assessor might look for in relation to the MCA. This allows comparison with relevant areas of their own practice. The following provides a summary of these indicators:

- Routine communication directly with service users "so that they understand their care, treatment and condition and any advice given".

- Communication adapted and delivered in a way that is accessible to our service users.

- Additional support (e.g., advocacy) implemented to help service users make decisions.

- Proactive and open involvement of significant others in care decisions when their support is required.

- Understanding of the MCA's relevance to consent and decision making by all staff.

- How service users are supported to make decisions.

- Assessment and documentation of a suspicion of incapacity.

- Best interests processes correctly and holistically followed.

- Explanation of how restraint is avoided or used in a proportionate way.

- Checking if decisions made on someone's behalf, that involve restrictions or restraint, might amount to a deprivation of liberty.

Health professionals may be particularly interested in guidance that is specific to their own professions. In many cases, such guidance is related to consent. The parallels in terms of providing adequate information in an accessible way are really helpful. And whilst consent is a broader concept than capacity, "Mental capacity has been argued to be the key component of consent to treatment" (Lamont et al., 2013, p. 685). Table 3.7 provides links to a few useful documents relating to the MCA from professional groups, with example quotes relating to good practice from each. Additionally, at the time of writing, the RCSLT position statement on the MCA is currently in production.

5 Practical tips on training health professionals to support decision making and assess capacity in line with the MCA

Professionals who work in safeguarding offices will commonly give the following advice: "Follow the MCA". Whilst this clearly means different things to different people, depending on their level of knowledge and confidence, the advice is a fundamentally sound place to start. When cases have become complex and advice is being sought, a process of problem solving has usually already begun. It is often the case, however, that this approach has not made full use of the MCA legislation. This legislation is designed to provide "a robust framework professionals can follow which should eradicate subjectivity of assessments and promote service user autonomy even if some choices pose a risk" (Marshall & Sprung, 2016, p.407). Although the legislation does not provide trainees with a bespoke script for each interaction, it does provide a framework. The forthcoming NICE SCIE guidance on decision making and mental capacity (due for publication June 2018) will provide further support.

   The following steps provide a suggested framework, based on the author's experience, that may be helpful when discussing assessment of decision making:

Step 1: Establish in your own mind what the decision is. When a service user presents with care or treatment needs, experienced clinicians will often use clinical reasoning to rapidly, and semi-automatically, move

Table 3.7 Extracts from published multidisciplinary guidance relating to supported decision making, capacity assessment, and obtaining consent.

Discipline	Links	Useful statements
General medicine	General Medical Council: Consent Guidance – Assessing Capacity Link: http://www.gmc-uk.org/guidance/ethical_guidance/consent_guidance_accessing_capacity.asp	"You must not assume that because a patient lacks capacity to make a decision on a particular occasion, they lack capacity to make any decisions at all, or will not be able to make similar decisions in the future." "If your assessment leaves you in doubt about the patient's capacity to make a decision, you should seek advice from…colleagues with relevant specialist experience, such as psychiatrists, neurologists, or speech and language therapists."
GPs	Royal College of General Practitioner: Mental Capacity Act Toolkit Link: https://www.bma.org.uk/advice/employment/ethics/mental-capacity/mental-capacity-toolkit	Try the following questions on eliciting carry-over of information: "What do you think this decision means? How will this decision affect you? Why do you think this decision needs to be made?" On weighing: "What will happen if you make this decision? What will happen if you do not make this decision?"
Surgeons	Royal College of Surgeons guidance on Consent Link: https://www.rcseng.ac.uk/standards-and-research/gsp/domain-3/3-5-1-consent/	"Recognise that seeking consent for surgical intervention is not merely the signing of a form. It is the process of providing the information that enables the patient to make a decision to undergo a specific treatment. Consent should be considered informed decision making, or informed request. It requires time, patience and clarity of explanation." "Ensure that the patient has sufficient time and information to make an informed decision. The specific timing and duration of the discussion should take into account the complexity and risks of the proposed procedure." "Where possible, you should provide written information to patients to enable them to reflect and confirm their decision. You should also provide advice on how they can obtain further information to understand the procedure and their condition. This can include information such as information leaflets, decision aids, websites and educational videos."
Emergency	The Royal College of Emergency Medicine Best Practice Guideline http://www.rcem.ac.uk/docs/RCEM%20Guidance/RCEM%20Mental%20Capacity%20Act%20in%20EM%20Practice%20-%20Feb%202017.pdf	"All Emergency Department (ED) doctors should understand the Mental Capacity Act (MCA) and be trained to be comfortable assessing a patient's capacity." On consultation with others: "Difficult decisions about a patient's capacity should be shared with a senior doctor."

Profession	Source	Guidance
Psychiatrists	Royal College of Psychiatrists: Capacity and The Mental Capacity Act Link: http://www.rcpsych.ac.uk/healthadvice/problemsdisorders/mentalcapacityandthelaw.aspx	On the time-specific nature of capacity and fluctuating capacity: "Capacity can change with time because your state of mind can change with time. An illness that interferes with your thinking can get better – at least for a while. An older person can become confused with a chest infection, so that they can't make many decisions properly. Their normal state of mind can return when the infection is treated and they can, again, make decisions in the way they normally would."
Psychologists	The British Psychological Society: Mental Capacity Act 2005 – Short Reference Guide for Psychologists and Psychiatrists Link: http://www.bps.org.uk/system/files/Public%20files/Policy/mental_capacity_act_2005_-_short_reference_guide_for_psychologists_and_psychiatrists%20REP47.pdf	On unwise decisions: "The law recognises the right of individuals to make unwise decisions. Such decisions might alert to the possibility of incapacity but they are NOT sufficient to determine a person's lack of capacity to make that specific decision."
Occupational Therapists	College of Occupational Therapists: Code of Ethics and Professional Conduct Link: https://www.rcot.co.uk/sites/default/files/CODE-OF-ETHICS-2015_0.pdf	On the conflict between paternalism and autonomy: "Where service users have mental capacity, they have a right to make informed choices and decisions about their future and the care and intervention that they receive...such choices should be respected, even when in conflict with professional opinion."
Physiotherapists	Chartered Society of Physiotherapists: Information Paper – Consent and Physiotherapy Practice www.csp.org.uk/sites/files/csp/secure/pd078consent2011_sep11_0.pdf	"Ensure that information is provided to patients in a way that is intelligible to them, in a place and manner where they are best able to understand and retain the information." "You should give information to patients in a balanced way. Where the evidence for the options under consideration is not equally balanced, you should inform the patients of all options and may offer your opinion as to the preferred option. You must not put pressure on the patient to accept your advice."
Social Workers	British Association of Social Workers / Brain Injury Social Work Group: Practice Guidance for Social Workers working with people with an acquired Brain Injury Link: http://cdn.basw.co.uk/upload/basw_123858-5.pdf	"Social workers are aware that breaking down information into discrete chunks, checking people have understood before moving on – and asking open questions about what has been understood are useful techniques. If there are significant speech and language difficulties a referral to a Speech and Language professional may well be essential and should be sought as part of the assessment process."

(Continued over)

Table 3.7 Extracts from published multidisciplinary guidance relating to supported decision making, capacity assessment, and obtaining consent.
(*Continued*)

Discipline	Links	Useful statements
Nurses	Royal College of Nursing: Principles of Consent – Guidance for Nursing Staff Link: https://www.rcn.org.uk/professional-development/publications/pub-006047	"If a person has capacity to make decisions independently then their decision is binding and the proposed examination, treatment, care or support cannot proceed, even if you think their decision is wrong."
CCGs/Trust Executives	Mental Capacity Act 2005: A Guide for Clinical Commissioning Groups and other commissioners of healthcare services on Commissioning for Compliance Link: https://www.england.nhs.uk/wp-content/uploads/2014/09/guide-for-clinical-commissioning.pdf	The MCA is rights legislation. It protects the rights of all service users to take as many decisions about themselves for as long as possible. It places on staff a duty to help service users make decisions for themselves.

through an assessment and management plan to respond to this need. Sharing the relevant parts of this process with the service user involves stating these thoughts aloud. Firstly, what is the issue, what are the care or treatments needed? Secondly, what are the options (even if there is only one treatment option there is almost invariably a second decision-making option – not doing anything at all)? If you can't summarize this process in your own head, you're not going to be able to help the service user to do so. Working through this process is also an essential part of the best interests' decision-making process and can be used to support that process at a later point if required.

Step 2: If you have had trouble working through Step 1, **make sure you're the right person to support the decision** in terms of your knowledge and expertise about the decision itself. If not, find someone who does or ensure that you are thoroughly briefed and supported by someone who does.

Step 3: **Establish how urgently the decision needs to be made**. Guidance within the MCA Code of Practice itself (Sec 2.9, Department of Constitutional Affairs, 2007) acknowledges that in urgent or emergency situations, healthcare professionals may have to make very quick use of the information available. In such cases, prioritizing life-saving intervention over further information gathering, or long-winded capacity assessment is completely appropriate.

Other decisions may allow a greater window of time, and an increased expectation that additional practicable steps to support the service user to make, or contribute substantially to making, their own decision will have been put in place. The case study below is an example which can be used to illustrate that even in some urgent cases (non-emergency), it is possible to provide comprehensive support.

Case Study 2 Applying the MCA in a complex and urgent case

A 69-year-old woman was admitted to Accident and Emergency with dizzy spells. Investigations revealed an underlying heart condition that would likely lead to sudden death from cardiac arrest if untreated. The insertion of a pacemaker would stabilize the condition and greatly reduce the risk of cardiac arrest occurring, almost certainly extending lifespan.

A senior doctor (Doctor A) from the treating team explained the recommendation to urgently fit a pacemaker and the risks of not doing so. The service user was adamant that she did not wish to proceed with the operation. The rationale for this decision appeared to be partly based on the fact that the service user had previously refused a pacemaker some years before and had subsequently remained well for several years. Additionally, the service user acknowledged a lifelong phobia of being 'cut' in the context of surgical procedures.

Doctor A discussed the service user's conversation and refusal with a medical colleague (Doctor B) raising concerns about the service user's wish to refuse a pacemaker and her ability to make a capacitous decision in this regard. Doctor B had a further conversation with the service user and felt the service user did have capacity to refuse, but acknowledged some uncertainty around this conclusion. As their conversations had not completely eliminated doubt regarding the service user's ability to understand the implications of a specific decision (acceptance or refusal of the pacemaker) Doctors A and B decided to explore the service user's history to check if they were missing anything relevant to the case and simultaneously made a referral to the MCA Practitioner in the Safeguarding Team for support.

The service user's history was reviewed. Now retired, she had worked as an office cleaner for 40 years. Following the death of her husband nine years before, she had no remaining family and was unable to identify next of kin. The terms 'learning difficulties' and 'anxiety' were included in her previous medical history. A previous discussion, recorded eight years earlier, relating to a recommendation for pacemaker insertion, was found. The service user clearly refused on this occasion also. It was also clear that the implications of not having the pacemaker at this earlier point were not imminently life threatening, and that the underlying heart condition had deteriorated considerably since then. A learning disability could not be confirmed. However, in terms of the two-stage test, observed difficulties relating to memory and planning in conversation supported a suspicion amongst all clinicians that the service user had some level of cognitive impairment. Additionally, the service user's cardiac condition made it difficult to exclude the possibility of ongoing risk of a reduced supply of oxygen to the brain. Finally, the impact of anxiety on the service user's ability to weigh and evaluate information was also considered.

The decision was made to try and provide additional support to the service user to make her own decision if possible, with the understanding that a best interests' decision-making process might result if attempts to support were unsuccessful. The steps taken were as follows.

An independent advocacy service was approached to see if a service user representative could be recruited but, having heard the details of the case, they felt that the urgency prevented this step from being taken and that the surgeon proposing the pacemaker should lead decision making around the service user's capacity to refuse (or accept) treatment and an appropriate course of action in the service user's best interests if capacity was found to be lacking.

The MCA Practitioner worked with two consultants to summarize the minimum key information relating to the risks and benefits or having, and not having, the operation. Prompts were integrated into the script to ensure the service user's processing of the key information was checked, and the reasons for any responses she provided requested. The information was presented to the service user, with back-up written information. Two hours of thinking time was then provided before the information was re-presented.

During interactions with the service user, she consistently communicated that she did not want the procedure. She was unable to give a clear reason for this but fear of being 'cut' was again implied. She reported understanding what the doctors had told her about the risks of not having the procedure but her ability to retain the information was inconsistent. The service user gave some indication that she had insight into suggested implications of refusing the procedure though, reporting that she was not overly concerned with the possibility of dying, as all those dear to her had already passed on. However, she appeared unable to consistently link highly increased risk of herself actually dying in the near future to not having the procedure. She consistently reported looking forward to attending a community group holiday in six months' time, and refuted the high likelihood that she would probably not be alive to attend it if the pacemaker was not fitted. She also repeatedly referred to earlier refusal of the pacemaker without adverse effects, but appeared unable to weigh the substantial deterioration in her heart condition that made the implications of the current decision different. She also reported enjoying life, particularly her thrice weekly sessions at the community group.

Following the interaction, the two consultants and the MCA practitioner discussed the attempts to support the service user's options and thoughts on her capacity to refuse the pacemaker. All agreed that, whilst she had been very clear in communicating her wishes and appeared to understand a key risk of her decision in isolation, it was not clear that she was able to demonstrate an ability to weigh and evaluate the information in the context of her own circumstances and future plans.

In moving to a best interests' decision, the urgent need for intervention, potentially to save life, removed the option of delaying the decision as a less restrictive option. The decision was made to proceed with insertion of the pacemaker, balancing the service user's feedback, information gained about their life, and the clinical risks. As part of the best interests' plan, psychological support was arranged for the service user prior to the procedure with a view to providing psychological aftercare following the procedure given the fact that the procedure was going ahead even though the service user had communicated that she did not want it to.

Three issues stand out in this case study. Firstly, even in complex and urgent cases, some degree of consultation is often possible, lending robustness to the decision-making process. Secondly, giving a service user the opportunity and time to explain their decision making can be crucial when judging their capacity and/or when considering what represents their best interests. Thirdly, it struck all the clinicians present that a few slight changes to the discussion might have resulted in a different conclusion being reached about the service user's capacity to consent. However, a decision had to be made, and made quickly, so the two-stage test was applied, and a carefully structured supported discussion used to clarify the difficult distinction between an unwise and an incapacitous decision. The decision maker consulted and a consensus-based best interests' decision was reached on the information available. The decision pathway was well documented to enable anyone reviewing the case to understand how and why the decision was reached.

Cases like this illustrate that whilst the MCA asks clinicians to use key principles to work fairly and systematically towards a decision, applying the legislation does not always equate to reaching a conclusion that is easy, unanimous, or comfortable for all those involved.

Step 4: Consider whether the decision relates to routine care and treatment or if this is something more serious. The legislation within the MCA infers a sliding scale, where the formality of supporting and then interrogating someone's capacity prior to decision making that affects them is proportionate to the seriousness of the decision being taken. As with urgency, there is a direct relationship between the seriousness of the decision and the extent of supportive steps and resources expected under the MCA.

Step 5: Know your 'service user'. Understanding a service user, with their own unique history, perspectives and background, requires a more holistic approach. Gathering a picture of the person's social, cultural, ethnic and religious and clinical background may provide key insights into the factors that might influence their decision making.

Medical history may also be examined at this point to establish, without prejudice, if there is "an impairment of the mind or brain, or is there some sort of disturbance affecting the way their mind or brain works" (MCA Code of Practice, 2007, p. 41). Table 3.8 gives examples of common clinical presentations that would fit this description.

Any such impairment or disturbance is not, itself, a reason to overturn the presumption of capacity. It may, though, be a trigger to finding out about the 'normal' cognition and communication function of the individual. Knowing who the service user has identified as significant or trusted others and asking them to provide supporting information can be helpful in this regard. Additionally, reviewing (or directly discussing) if other members of the MDT, (including GPs and external providers) or significant others are aware of any issues with thinking or communicating can help highlight specific needs or issues (see step 7 for further details).

This is also the time to find out if the service user has made any advanced decisions or nominated a Lasting Power of Attorney for Health and Welfare decisions. Not only might these steps to 'know your service user' help optimise interactions with them, but should they later be found unable to make a decision for themselves, the information gathered could be invaluable to the decision-making process that occurs on their behalf.

Step 6: Take a staged approach to consent. This will tell you more about your service user and their needs. A supportive and enabling approach to gaining consent is likely to provide invaluable information about the

Table 3.8 Issues that may be associated with an impairment / disturbance of mind or brain

Delirium, overt confusion, sepsis or drowsiness secondary to illness
Acquired neurological injury or degenerative, progressive process, for example:
Head injury / TBI, Stroke,
Brain tumour / Space occupying lesion
Seizures,
Encephalitis, Some cases of Multiple Sclerosis,
Some cases of Parkinson's disease
Symptoms of drug or alcohol use
Mental health disturbance
Learning disability
Dementia
Endocrine disturbance
Persistently reduced GCS
Hypoxia

kind of support a service user may require in order to process a particular decision. The two-stage test can reveal a potential reason to question presumed capacity and, most importantly, give the service user a rounded initial opportunity to understand, recall and weigh information about a decision, and then communicate a preference, long before any more formal process might be needed. The approach outlined in Table 3.9 (adapted from Joshi, 2015, itself adapted from Douglas & Fiske, 2008) is a suggested approach to such an opening discussion.

If it is not possible to have such a discussion (as outlined in Table 3.9), or if attempts fail, and the need to take the decision needs to be delayed to allow for further support, then the hope is that moving through these stages will have provided valuable information. This would include obtaining information about the types of difficulties a person is having that need problem solving – including the identification of appropriate support measures or tools in order to move forward. This discussion is also likely to provide information about the second element of the two-stage test: whether any impairment or disturbance of mind or brain appears to be impacting on a person's ability to make a specific decision at a specific time. This would raise a possible reason to doubt or overturn presumption of capacity and, if further practicable steps to support fail, trigger initiation of a formal capacity assessment.

Step 7: Ask yourself again: Is additional support required? Table 3.10 provides a checklist of basic additional support requirements that will need consideration before a capacity assessment takes place.

Table 3.9 A staged approach to gaining consent.

Introduction
Establish what is already understood
Explain the nature of the clinical condition
Outline treatment options
Explain risks and benefits
Check what has been understood
Invite further questions
Confirm the preferred treatment option
Obtain confirmed consent

Moving beyond 'the basics', holistic case history taking and provisional discussions may have flagged up a need for professional support in interactions relating to decision making. This may involve one or multiple professionals. If time allows, the emphasis should be on recruiting support early enough in the process to ensure trusting relationships are developed with appropriate professionals who can help the person work towards making their own decision (see Case Study 3.)

Case Study 3: MDT working together to maximize capacity

A 75-year-old woman was admitted with severe pain in her groin. Investigations were undertaken and the resulting clinical recommendation was for a further, invasive procedure. The primary benefits of the procedure were that the intervention would almost immediately stop the pain and would also prevent the underlying cause of pain from spreading (a spread which would, at some stage, lead to a further and possibly serious deterioration in health). The drawbacks were related to the general risks of surgery, and the fact that the surgery would result in permanent physical changes to the service users' appearance and sexual function.

Table 3.10 A checklist of basic additional support requirements that will need consideration before a capacity assessment takes place.

Additional support	Yes/No	Comments
Does the individual need to wear glasses during the discussions?		
Does the individual need hearing aids and, if so, are they available and working?		
Does the individual need an interpreter (if non-English speaker or if English is a second language and first language is preferred)?		
Is an alternative environment required for discussions and assessment, e.g.m to minimize distractions?		
Does the individual want the involvement of family or friends in the decision-making process?		
If the answer is 'yes' to the above, are the identified family members/friends available and willing to take part in discussions?		
Is an advocate required to support the individual?		
Are printed or image-based resources available and useful in helping the individual reflect on the information over a period of time?		
If the answer is 'yes' to the above, have these been provided?		

The woman's behaviour was very difficult to manage on the ward. She presented as verbally and physically aggressive at times and typically refused examination. A delirium of uncertain cause was identified, and service user history and psychological assessment were suggestive of Korsakoff's dementia. Psychological assessment also suggested marked difficulties with working memory and low mood but otherwise above average intelligence. In conversation, it appeared difficult for the service user to follow lengthy or complex information but she was able to speak fluently and articulately. Conversations relating to the medical recommendations proved difficult to undertake. When the service user built a rapport with one key team member she eventually reported a long history of sexual abuse. She reported that her history made her very reluctant to allow examination and she was also very opposed to the idea of surgical intervention. On more than one occasion, she clearly reported a desire to die rather than have surgical intervention and would certainly want to die if physical changes were forced upon her against her will. Psychiatric review resulted in the recommendation of 1:1 supervision by a registered mental health nurse. Attempts to discuss this further and to consider the implications of doing nothing were typically curtailed by the service user, who was also becoming increasingly frustrated by her hospital admission and asking to leave. The service user's relationships with staff appeared variable, depending on the staff member, and she claimed she felt overwhelmed by the information she was receiving from different members of staff and felt trapped in the hospital (of note, a DoLs was initiated during the admission).

Full assessment of her capacity was challenging due to the difficulty of engaging her in extended conversation (she would typically ask to discontinue the conversation). Various opinions about her decision-making capacity were recorded, alongside recommendations from a variety of different team members relating to behavioural management and potential discharge planning. In a service user with complex mental and physical health needs there were multiple stakeholders and advisors all making recommendations relating to care in their area of expertise.

The case was referred to the Trust's MCA practitioner. A case conference was arranged, attended by key members of the MDT. The initial aims of the conference were to arrive at a best interests' decision but, during the meeting, it became clear more work needed to be done to support the service user in making a decision in relation to surgery. To optimize the service user's ability to contribute to discussions the following supports and least restrictive options were put in place:

- The pain management team were involved to improve management of the service user's acute discomfort.

- Same-sex nurses were employed and a rota involving a small number of nurses (prioritizing those with whom the service user had establish rapport) was put in place.

- The nurses supported the service user to have time off the ward in a wheelchair to smoke cigarettes.

- All non-essential nursing interventions were stopped.

- A consistent approach to communicating the risks and benefits of having and not having surgery were scripted, with advice from the MCA practitioner and psychologist on tailoring the information into manageable chunks and maintaining a neutral tone that avoided steering the service user but provided clarity around all implications.

- Open questions were integrated into this script to ensure the service user's voice and reasoning were elicited.

- The surgeon responsible for undertaking the relevant procedure revisited conversations with the service user regularly, supported by a specialist nurse.

- A written copy of the information was provided to the service user (to aid retention) and to key staff (to ensure handover was consistent).

With the service user's consent, her primary next of kin was included in the circulation of this script, and also spoke about it with the service user. However, as the next of kin felt she would be unable to act as an objective representative on the service user's behalf (because of the strength of her opinion that the service user should have the surgery), an external paid advocate was employed to provide the service user with a neutral source of support.

Following improved pharmacological management of the service user's pain and five days of consistent orientation the service user began to demonstrate carryover of key information and conversations. This change suggested she was better able to understand, recall and weigh key information. At this point ,the service user maintained that she was genuinely (and understandably) struggling to make such a difficult decision. The MCA had been fully explained to the service user at this stage, who understood that if she could not decide, a best interests' process might commence but that her wishes would very much be part of that process, and that her independent advocate could act as an IMCA to support the process. In the first instance, she asked for more time to reach a decision. This was provided as the least restrictive option. Nine days after treatment of her pain had been optimized, and key information had been consistently discussed, and the service user had received two visits from the independent advocate, the service user made the decision to proceed with the surgery. She was jointly assessed by the lead clinician and a supporting member of the team to have capacity to make this decision. What was also noticeable over this period was that the service user's behaviour on the ward improved dramatically and her ability to consent to her ongoing admission also returned.

Post-surgery the service user presented as pain free and she thanked the lead clinician for allowing her to come to the decision herself.

Key thoughts:

- Management of the case improved when key staff sat down and planned a coordinated approach.

- The clinical lead took a genuine interest in addressing the psychosocial aspects of the service user's care as well as the clinical needs.

- The team were able to work together to address reversible issues impacting on decision making representing a constructive use of the least restrictive option.

- The team worked together to tailor and improve consistency in the delivery of information to meet the service user's cognitive needs.

- Having an aim in place around decision making and a plan to achieve it provided a rationale in the face of daily discharge pressures.

- The delay in deciding whether or not to proceed with surgery allowed the service user to recover to a point where she was able to independently make a capacitous decision. Had the service user not been supported, her objections may have continued, and the next step could arguably have been a Court of Protection referral, a process that would most likely have been stressful and time consuming for all involved and almost certainly resulted in an increased length of stay.

Luff and Volkmer provide a useful overview about how members of the MDT can provide support to a person who may lack capacity (see Chapter 6 in Volkmer, 2016). SLTs can provide a wide range of support to make decision making more accessible to service users, and to making core processes that form part of the MCA more accessible to the MDT. Volkmer (2016) summarizes some of the different roles SLTs can take on but, broadly speaking, they can offer expertise on adapting communication to an appropriate level for a service user who has any kind of disturbance of their speech intelligibility, understanding and expression (of spoken, written and/or picture-based information) or compensating for cognitive difficulties that may be impacting on communication. An SLT can provide information that can guide the interactions of others, direct support for such service users to process information relevant to a particular decision, communicate preferences or opinions, or may be involved in directly assessing a person's capacity to make decisions when acquired communication impairments are impacting on interactions. See Chapter 3 of Volkmer (2016) for a more in-depth description.

If there is a known mental health issue, including dementia, which may be impacting on interactions and decision making, a psychiatrist is well placed to provide support. If cognitive issues are felt to be impacting, then psychology or occupational therapy support can be of help. Psychologists may also be able to support teams when the process of decision making causes disagreement between professionals, service users, and significant others. Occupational therapists have considerable expertise in supporting individuals to understand risks relating to discharge, based on real-world assessments that look at a person's likely ability to manage daily activities of necessity and choice, through self-care, to accessing the community and financial management. Social workers may routinely conduct capacity assessments as part of their role, and have a key role in identifying living options following a service user's discharge.

In summary, the MDT offers a comprehensive resource for service users who need additional support. That support may take many forms, including joint sessions with a service user, assessment leading to the provision of practical guidance for optimizing interactions, directly supporting capacity assessment, or providing crucial information to be considered as part of a best interests' decision.

Step 8: Provide enhanced support: Effectively, this stage amounts to revisiting stage 6 but with additional structure and resources. Once the barriers to information processing are clearer, the process of introducing oneself and one's role, establishing baseline understanding, explaining the clinical condition, outlining the decision options (and associated risks and benefits) and then moving between checking what has been understood, and attempting to fill in any gaps, begins again. It should be added here, that at this point a healthcare professional may not always have time on their side. The support of others may be limited or unavailable within a given timeframe. But this does not mean that further steps to optimizing interactions focused on decision making are not possible. Table 3.11 summarizes the approach to support outlined in Step 6, adding practical descriptions of what enhanced support might look like. Further guidance and discussion around making information accessible is provided by Jayes (in Volkmer, 2016) and in Chapter 6 of this book.

Step 9: Assessment of decision-making capacity and documentation A holistic capacity assessment should evolve from the steps provided above, representing the final, optimally-supported version of a decision specific discussion. There are several proformas available to guide documentation (Jayes & Palmer, 2014, is a good example, shown in Volkmer, 2016, pp. 130-131).

However an assessment is written up, the following detail is recommended:

1. Who was present for the assessment

2. The specific decision

Table 3.11 Providing enhanced support.

Stage	Contents of each stage	Making the information accessible
Planning	Know the decision. Know the key information needed to help someone make a decision. Know/agree the threshold you would expect someone to meet to demonstrate capacity. Prepare some simple questions or conversation 'starters' to allow the service user to engage in an introductory conversation with you.	Use simple language Use short sentences Avoid jargon or technical language Provide one piece of information at a time
Introduction	State who you are and the purpose of your visit.	Provide information in a logical order
Build rapport and a reliable method of communication	Use prepared questions/topics. Apply the 'Tips for making information accessible' and note effective strategies. NB: This itself may require a session or number of sessions.	Make sure each point makes sense in isolation Go slow – allow extra time for a person to process each point
Establish what is already understood	Ask the service user why they are in the healthcare setting.	Repeat and re-phrase
Explain the nature of the clinical condition	Clearly outline the decision to be made. Attempt to clarify and explain anything the service user does not understand. Provide a timeframe, if possible, of when the decision should ideally be made.	Use colour images to support key information (photos, without 'busy' backgrounds)
Outline treatment options	Offer key information about each option. Include the option of no treatment/intervention.	
Explain risks and benefits and implications	Explain serious or common risks. One by one, cover the key risks and benefits of inaction also. Explain the likely implications of the decision on the person and those around them.	

Check what has been understood	Ask questions as you go along. Ask the service user to summarize what they have heard so far. Correct any misunderstandings, then ask questions, elicit summary again.	If providing options for an individual to choose from OR using only Yes/No questions, cross-check responses for consistency (e.g., ask the same questions more than once to see if you get the same response)
Invite further questions	Encourage the service user to take the opportunity to ask questions or raise concerns.	
Try to confirm preferred treatment option	Ask the service user for their preference. Explore why a person has made this decision (their rationale may provide crucial information allowing a healthcare professional to distinguish between an unwise versus an incapacitous decision. Ask the person if they need more time, information or support.	Repeat and rephrase if you see any signs that something hasn't been understood. Ensure written information is available and that it: – is written in a large font
Reflect on the session and, if feasible, plan further session of support	If, after the above steps have been taken, the service user has not been able to make a capacitous decision, consider if further adaptations and additional support sessions are indicated and plan/schedule these accordingly, repeating the steps above.	– is well-spaced – has a small number of words per page **You may require the support of the relevant professional, e.g., SLT/Psychology

3. The key information relevant to the decision

4. The impairment or disturbance of mind or brain (and consideration of whether this is temporary or reversible)

5. How each part of the functional test of decision-making ability was assessed (understanding, recall, weighing and communication of key information)

6. The support in place to help the service user meet the demands of each stage of the functional test

7. Key examples of the service user's responses (recording exactly what was seen or heard)

8. Link service user's responses to each stage of the functional test – with comments on whether or not the response equates to a demonstration of ability to fulfil each stage of the functional test.

9. A conclusion about the service user's capacity to make the decision.

Step 10: Best Interests Advising an approach to effectively supporting best interests' decision making arguably requires a chapter in its own right. However, if clinicians have implemented the first three principles of the MCA before arriving at this stage, then a large amount of the groundwork will already be in place. Support provided to the service user and discussion of the decision or decisions to be made, what the service user's preferences are, and why the service user has reached that decision should all be factored in to a best interests' decision.

Establishing the nature and extent of a service user's social network, as part of the support and capacity assessment process, should include exploration of advanced provisions for decision making (e.g., Lasting Power of Attorney for health and welfare, Court Appointed Deputy, recorded advanced decision). Such investigation might identify a best interests' decision maker outside of the team of health and social care professionals working with the person. Any potential need for an IMCA or independent advocate should have been identified by this point too.

If no such advanced provisions are present, the decision maker in relation to the service user's capacity to make a particular decision, is likely to maintain their position as lead decision maker in a best interests' decision. One of their first roles may be to explain to the next of kin how the best interests process works, and clearly set out the role of friends or family in providing crucial supporting information whilst making it clear that that the person making the final decision about care and treatment will be a clinician. Whoever takes the lead should also make use of the information and opinions gathered during the decision-making process to reach a decision on the service user's behalf. There will always be situations where a decision is so urgent it has to be made quickly, and sometimes unilaterally, with the information available. Explicit guidance to include the MDT in **all** best interests' decision making is lacking in the code of practice. However, in most cases, consultation and building consensus remains key. Ultimately, the decision maker must be able to account for why any consultation was considered either impractical or inappropriate.

Finally, a best interests' decision should be reached, in most cases, by considering and giving equal credence to the blend of clinical risks and benefits, the service user's personal wishes, values and beliefs, and the key social and psychological factors that the service user might take into account. Figure 3.2 demonstrates how these issues may overlap and impact on decision making.

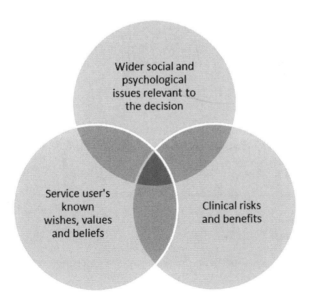

Figure 3.2 The key considerations that should overlap when reaching a best interests' decision.

6 Working together and managing conflict: Navigating a consensus approach to implementing the MCA

Barriers to effective implementation of the MCA may exist at strategic or operational levels. Variable understanding of the Act may interplay with established hierarchies in the team which, if poorly managed, can lead to conflict. Trainees may find that applying the MCA competes with discharge pressures, and an understandable desire to avoid disagreement with a service user, family members and colleagues. Any of the stakeholders involved in a service user's care and treatment may disagree about a service user's ability to make their own decisions, the type and extent of support that might enable them to make a particular decision, what is in their best interest, and even proportionate use of restrictions and restraint to facilitate the delivery of treatment in their best interest.

It is not the individual clinician's responsibility to meet all these challenges. Table 3.12 provides some suggestions and practical approaches that can support organizations, teams and individuals in this process.

Table 3.12 Practical approaches to supporting consensus based approach to the MCA.

Strategic level	The organization should have a dedicated policy relating to local application of the MCA.
	The organization should have an agreed training framework for the MCA covering all service user-facing staff.
	Senior/key decision makers should be supported to access higher level scenario-based training to effectively support resolution of escalated cases.
	Practice in relation to the MCA should be widely and regularly audited, with teams actively involved in audits to support case-based learning.
	Effective implementation of the MCA should be supported at a senior level in an organization.
	Regular awareness raising around the MCA should be in place.
Operational level (systems, processes and resources)	There should be documentation in place from the point of admission and as part of medical, nursing and therapeutic care plans which capture difficulties relating to thinking and communication that may impact on decision making.
	Difficulties with care and treatment decision making should be routinely discussed during MDT meetings/board rounds.
	Reference to whether serious care or treatment decisions are being made with the service user's agreement and consent, or in their best interests should be routinely included as part of team discussions.

	Decision-making flowcharts related to supported decision making, capacity assessment, and best interests' decision making should be used to guide related discussions, assessments, family meetings and proxy decision making.
	Use of the MCA should be embedded into local training programmes. Case studies relevant to the clinical area in question should be included.
	Information tailored to staff, service users and families relating to the MCA should be available in accessible formats.
	Pro-formas to support capacity assessments and best interests' decisions should be available to help guide staff, who require such support, and optimize their documentation.
	Referral to other specialties (e.g., SLTs, OTs and Psychology) to support decision making should be routine in cases where known cognitive or communication difficulties are present.
	Independent advice/second opinions should be routinely sought when disagreements in relation to the MCA occur (e.g., local experts/Champions, Internal Safeguarding team, local authority DoLs/safeguarding team, local legal team, local advocacy or IMCA service).
	SLT/OT/ Psychology teams should promote their skillset in relation to supporting information processing in people with cognitive and communication difficulties and explicitly link these skills to issues around mental capacity.
Individual level	Discussions with service users to establish if they understand why they are receiving a particular care or treatment action should be routine.
	For more complex decisions, explaining how the MCA works, to service users and to family members, should be part of routine practice.
	Individual clinicians should understand their own role and the role of others in relation to a particular treatment decision (i.e., who is the decision maker, who is supporting access to information, who is providing additional information and feedback that will support the process).
	Individuals should know how to escalate, and who to escalate to, when disagreements in relation to the MCA occur.
	Senior individuals in the team should recognize the need to consult widely with others involved in a service user's care: particularly when reaching decisions about a service user's capacity to consent/or what is in their best interests in serious medical treatment or discharge decisions.
	Individual clinicians should routinely document the decision pathway that led to their conclusion about a service user's capacity or the course of action considered to be in the service user's best interests.

Summary

As mentioned in the introduction to this chapter, SLTs are well placed to train other professionals in adapting and shaping communicative interactions. SLTs are also skilled in identifying individuals who may have difficulty making some decisions, and supporting them to do so. In order to do this, and train others to do so, SLTs need to have a thorough understanding of the MCA itself.

SLTs may also benefit from a broader understanding of why practice relating to the MCA can be so variable. This can expose deeply entrenched and established approaches to service user care that may be at odds with the MCA's enabling approach. It is valuable to understand the common pitfalls in practice relating to the MCA. Once these are openly discussed, trainees (including SLTs) can better understand the perspectives and needs of their service users. The MCA presents a framework against which practice can be audited and improved, ultimately ensuring a fair and accessible opportunity for all service users to participate equally in decision making about their own health and welfare where possible.

Additional resources

There are an increasing number of resources available to support understanding and implementation of the MCA. The following are some particularly useful links and resources when training others.

- Social Care Institute of Excellence (SCIE) website: https://www.scie.org.uk/mca/ A repository for a wealth of information relating to all things MCA, with links to case studies, videos, information guides and useful networks.

- The SCIE website includes tools and resources specific to professionals working in healthcare settings: https://www.scie.org.uk/mca-directory/mca-tailored-for-you/health/index.asp

- MCA Competency Framework: Produced by the University of Bournemouth's National Centre for Post Qualifying Social Work and Professional Practice, it provides an accessible overview of the key elements of the MCA and how they should be applied. Suggests a framework for training and competency development by professional grouping.   http://www.ncpqsw.com/publications/national-mental-capacity-act-competency-framework/

- 39 Essex Chambers Mental Capacity Newsletter: Provides accessible updates on cases involving the MCA, with interpretation and implications for case law. http://www.39essex.com/tag/mental-capacity-newsletter/

- MCA code of Practice: Essential reading as a source document to guide best practice: https://www.gov.uk/government/publications/mental-capacity-act-code-of-practice

References

Acquired Brain Injury and Mental Capacity Act Interest Group (2014). Acquired Brain Injury and Mental Capacity. Recommendations for Action following the House of Lords Select Committee Post-Legislative Scrutiny Report into the Mental Capacity Act: Making the Abstract Real. http://www.mentalcapacitylawandpolicy.org.uk/wp-content/uploads/2014/10/DoH-MCA-ABI-17-09-14.pdf

Atwal, A., McIntyre, A., & Wiggett, C. (2011). Risks with older adults in acute care settings: UK occupational therapists' and physiotherapists' perceptions of risk associated with discharge and professional practice. *Scandinavian Journal of Caring Sciences*, 26, 381–393.

Currie, L. MCA/DoLs Manager at Shropshire County Council, 2016, Presentation and notes from session at the National Mental Capacity Act Forum, UCL, 2016.

Department for Constitutional Affairs (2007). The Mental Capacity Act 2005 Code of Practice. London: The Stationery Office. https://www.gov.uk/government/publications/mental-capacity-act-code-of-practice

England and Wales High Court (Family Division) Mrs B vs an NHS Trust [2002] EWHC 429 (fam) http://www.bailii.org/ew/cases/EWHC/Fam/2002/429.html

England and Wales Court of Protection PH v A Local Authority [2011] EWCOP 1704 (30 June 2011) http://www.bailii.org/ew/cases/EWCOP/2011/1704.html

England and Wales Court of Protection, King's College Hospital NHS Foundation Trust v C [2015] EWCOP 80, [2015] MHLO 125 http://www.bailii.org/ew/cases/EWCOP/2015/80.html

England and Wales Court of Protection, Briggs v Briggs (by his litigation friend, the Official Solicitor) and others [2016] EWCOP http://www.bailii.org/ew/cases/EWCOP/2016/53.html

Gough, M. & Kerlin, L. (2012). Limits of the Mental Capacity Act training for residential care homes. *The Journal of Adult Protection*, 14(6), 271–279.

HM Government (2016). The National Mental Capacity Forum, Chair's Annual Report https://www.gov.uk/government/publications/national-mental-capacity-forum-chairs-annual-report-2016

Herring, J. (2009). Losing it? Losing what? The law and dementia., *Child and Family Law Quarterly*, 3.

House of Lords (2014). *Mental Capacity Act 2005: Post Legislative Scrutiny*. London: House of Lords.

Joshi, N. (2015). Assessments of service users' capacity to consent to treatment. *Learning Disability Practice*, 18(5), 34-35.

Lamont, S., Jeon, Y-H., & Chiarella, M. (2013a). Health-care professionals' knowledge, attitudes and behaviours relating to patient capacity to consent to treatment: An integrative review. *Nursing Ethics*, 20(6), 684-707

Lamont, S., Jeon, Y-H., & Chiarella, M. (2013b). Assessing patient capacity to consent to treatment: An integrative review of instruments and tools. *Journal of Clinical Nursing*, 22, 2387-2403.

Marshall, H. & Sprung, S. (2016a). Community nurses' knowledge, confidence and experience of the Mental Capacity Act in practice. *British Journal of Community Nursing*, 21(12). doi.org/10.12968/bjcn.2016.21.12.615

Marshall, H. & Sprung, S. (2016b). The Mental Capacity Act: A review of the current literature. *British Journal of Community Nursing*, 21(8), 406-410.

Murphy, G.H. (2006). *Assessment of Capacity in Adults: Interim Guidance for Psychologists*. London: British Psychological Society.

NHS England. Mental Capacity Act 2005. A Guide for Clinical Commissioning Groups and Other Commissioners of Healthcare Services on Commissioning for Compliance, April 2014.

Phair, L. & Manthorpe, J. (2012). The use of the Mental Capacity Act among hospital patients:Findings from a case study of one Acute Hospital Trust in England. *The Journal of Adult Protection*, 14(6), 259-270.

Volkmer, A. (2016). *Dealing with Capacity and Other Legal Issues with Adults with Acquired Neurological Conditions – A Resource for Speech and Language Therapists*. Guildford: J & R Press.

Wilner, P., Bridle, J., Price, V., Dymond, S., & Lewis, G. (2013). What do NHS staff learn from training on the Mental Capacity Act (2005)? *Legal and Criminological Psychology*, 18, 83-101.

Wilson, E., Seymour, J.E., & Perkine, P. (2010) Working with the Mental Capacity Act: Findings from specialist palliative and neurological settings. *Palliative Medicine*, (4), 396-402.

4 Working in care homes and other extended care environments

Rachel Daly

> "Where, after all, do universal human rights begin? In small places, close to home – so close and so small that they cannot be seen on any map of the world. Yet they are the world of the individual person ... Unless these rights have meaning there, they have little meaning anywhere." Eleanor Roosevelt

Introduction

This chapter explores what is meant by extended care environments, the people who live, work and visit there, and how they work with statutory care services provided by social care, the National Health Service (NHS) and other services. In 2011, an inquiry was conducted into the quality of healthcare for older people in care homes (Gladman & Bowman, 2012). The NHS support available to care homes was found to be unacceptably variable and often of poor quality. The report proposed the integration of health, social and care home leadership. It suggested that they work with statutory regulators and service user advocacy groups to find solutions that they have been unable to achieve alone.

The population living in extended care settings is diverse. Those affected by the Mental Capacity Act (MCA, 2005) include people with a wide range of cognitive impairments including dementia, learning disabilities, and acquired brain injuries amongst others. Here we are focusing on people living with dementia as their number vastly outweighs any other group and many of their issues in relation to the MCA will be similar, and thus transferable, to those experienced by other groups.

The case studies included in this chapter are anonymized but based on real people. They are designed so that you can reflect, debate and discuss your thoughts and feelings either alone or with a colleague or your team. There are no 'right answers' and you may react differently to your colleagues depending on your professional background and experience. Some possible answers and outcomes are offered as guidance.

This chapter is designed to:

- Explore what extended care environments are and how they work with community and hospital healthcare services
- Understand the people who live, work and visit extended care environments and the support they might need
- Examine the context of the MCA in extended care settings
- Discuss roles and relationships: Capacity and decision making
- Identify the role of the speech and language therapist (SLT) in supporting residents, staff and care partners in extended care settings
- Offer you an opportunity to reflect on MCA assessment case studies.

Having a robust understanding of the above, and reflecting on the case studies provided, will support you in delivering training on the MCA to professionals who work in extended care environments.

Extended care environments

'Extended care environments' are communal residential settings with onsite care provision; they include supported living, care villages and extra care housing as well as the more traditional care homes with and without nursing. They are all registered, regulated and inspected by the Care Quality Commission (CQC) in the UK. Indicators for good quality of care include (amongst others) person-centred care, privacy, equality and dignity, safeguarding and safety, adequate nutrition and suitably qualified staff (see http://www.cqc.org.uk/what-we-do/how-we-do-our-job/fundamental-standards for a full list of the fundamental standards).

This chapter focuses predominantly on care homes. However, they provide only a proportion of the extended care in the UK, with care villages and extra care housing becoming increasingly popular for older people and those living with a cognitive impairment. Supported living has long been favoured by learning disability services as providing optimum care. This option offers smaller, more intimate services that can be tailored to individual needs since large care institutions closed in the late 20th century. Supported living could also provide optimum person-centred care for many older people living with dementia. Unfortunately, this is not a viable option, either financially or logistically, in view of the anticipated increase in the European population of people over 65; set to almost double between 2010 and 2050.

Many care homes provide good quality person-centred care but they work within constraints of communal living. Meals are largely served at specified times and many activities organized to suit the many rather than the few. This is not true of all homes, and increasingly kitchen areas are open to residents, families and staff so that they can make toast or sandwiches whenever they please. Care staff and activity coordinators in some homes are also able to play games or undertake sensory activities with individuals on a rotational basis or based on individual need. For most care homes the days of bingo in the lounge being the highlight of the week are long gone.

Care home placements are normally funded in one of four ways: privately; social care; NHS continuing care; or a combination of social care and NHS, or social care and private 'top-up' funding (other combinations are available!). A typical care home bed may cost from as little as £800 to as much as £1500+ per week. The impact of care home funding on care delivery is far reaching. People living in care homes are not always entitled to NHS services. Many GPs argue that visiting care homes is not part of the General Medical Services (GMC) contract, and as such request additional payment to visit care homes. Health and social care commissioners may also place limitations on services that are available to care home residents. It is worth being aware of this age-old argument (which rages on) when you discuss what you can and cannot offer service users in care homes.

The care home workforce

The skill mix and number of staff in health and social care are considered to be determinants of the quality and efficiency of care. To understand the challenges faced by healthcare professionals visiting people living in a care home environment, it is important to understand and contextualize some of the workforce issues and the resident population. For example:

- The NHS employs about 1.4 million people, 48% of whom are highly educated and professionally qualified. Most care homes are considered to come under social care. Social care employs about 1.6 million people, less than 20% of whom are professionally qualified.
- NHS hospitals have about 150,000 beds. Care homes have around 450,000 beds.

The health service is therefore obviously much better staffed, which would seem to make sense due to the acute nature of the care provided in hospital beds. Yet anyone who has visited a care home recently will testify that the residents are increasingly incredibly frail with multiple long-term physical and mental health conditions; many are also receiving end-of-life care (Bunn et al., 2014; Goodman, Amador, Elmore, Machen, & Mathie, 2013).

There is no minimum staff-to-resident ratio in care homes. The quality, level and amount of training care home staff receive (beyond basic statutory and mandatory training) is largely dependent on the (care provider) organization.

The majority of care home staff are poorly paid and work long hours in sometimes challenging conditions.

Care home staff care for the frailest and most vulnerable people in our society. This workforce demonstrate knowledge and skills relevant to person-centred care that far surpasses that delivered in hospital settings (Care Quality Commission, 2014).

What this staff group does best is care! Meeting the care needs of this vulnerable group of people is time-consuming and complex. Many care home staff know the current and ongoing values, priorities and needs of their long-term residents as well as the residents' families. These staff can sometimes recognize small inferences made long after language is lost for people living with dementia. A greater emphasis is required on the important role that they play in supporting everyday decision making, as well as providing for physical care needs.

Many care home staff are aware of the need for services to be person-led, not just person-centred, and do whatever they can to ensure that the voice of the residents is included. These care staff are capable of delivering excellent dementia care. Research suggests that personal communication characteristics are as, if not more, important than dementia training (Clarke, 2004; Handley, Bunn, & Goodman, 2017). Many care home managers now put a greater emphasis on personal traits rather than traditional academic job requirements when employing staff and many good care homes include residents on their interview panel.

Given the volume and complexity of their workload it is unsurprising that care staff need support from a wide range of community healthcare professionals. These may include community nurses, podiatrists, SLTs, pharmacists, physiotherapists, occupational therapists, opticians, GPs and dentists amongst others. Each profession has its own valuable expertise to offer, depending on the needs of the individual resident and their fluctuating health needs.

Care home residents

Approximately 450,000 people live in care homes in the UK (Demos, 2014) and in excess of 70% of them are thought to have dementia or significant memory problems (Prince et al., 2014). The care home population has changed dramatically in the last decade or so; in part because people are able to remain at home and maintain their independence for longer. Thus, the care home population has become increasingly complex and frail.

Care home admission is often delayed until a health or social care (family) crisis occurs. Such crises may include a fractured hip following a fall, or family members no longer managing. This type of emergency admission is challenging for anyone forced into such a situation. For many it involves loss of a home, feelings of abandonment and changes to their standards of living. For some, it also includes the loss of a partner. For people living with dementia this may be coupled with additional disorientation causing distress and further confusion.

People living with dementia and their families are increasingly reliant on long-term residential care as the effects of dementia progress and daily care needs rise. Dementia care has increased in care home environments by about 20% in the UK in the last decade (Matthews et al., 2013). Almost 60% of people requiring dementia care are in residential homes with no onsite nursing provision (Prince et al., 2014). It is widely recognized that this population may need support and assistance with decisions about their day-to-day health and care (Department for Constitutional Affairs, 2007; Legislation.gov.uk, 2014).

The MCA in extended care environments

The ability to make a certain decision at a given time can be affected by physical, emotional, spiritual and environmental stimuli and therefore has the potential to affect anyone at any time. Prior to the implementation of the MCA in 2007 the law relating to people who lacked capacity was "fragmented, complex and out of date" (The Law Commission, 1991), and did not offer legal protection for people lacking capacity. Even after the MCA was passed in 2005 further challenges were identified in the HL v UK [2005] 'Bournewood' case which led to the Deprivation of Liberty Safeguards (2007) being appended to the MCA.

Many health and social care practitioners see the MCA (2005) as presenting issues of its own. The legal principles and the MCA Code of Practice (2007) offer useful instruction and guidance regarding its application. However, health and care staff sometimes feel the need to undertake and document mental capacity assessments where someone has an impairment of the 'mind or brain' (despite the individual clearly demonstrating capacity), as 'proof' of capacity. This may be due to poor experience of punitive safeguarding processes and could be seen to offer 'protection' to the care professional and the individual in question. However, it clearly contravenes Principle 1 of the MCA (presumption of capacity). An assessment should only be undertaken if there is reason to doubt the mental capacity of the individual in question. The 'protection imperative' is discussed below.

The five key principles of the MCA must always be applied in undertaking any mental capacity assessment to ensure that an individual's needs are respected and met appropriately whilst also ensuring that the law is implemented and the legal process followed. The Act creates an assurance framework for individuals who lack capacity, their care partners and for care providers to work within.

Table 4.1 The principles of the MCA (2005).

Principle 1	Presumption of capacity: "A person must be assumed to have capacity unless it is established that he lacks capacity"
Principle 2	Maximizing involvement: "A person is not to be treated as unable to make a decision unless all practical steps to help him to do so have been taken without success"
Principle 3	Unwise decisions: "A person is not to be treated as unable to make a decision merely because he makes an unwise decision"
Principle 4	Best interests: "An act done, or decision made, under this Act for or on behalf of a person who lacks capacity must be done, or made, in his best interests"
Principle 5	Less restriction: "Before the act is done, or the decision is made, regard must be had to whether the purpose for which it is needed can be effectively achieved in a way that is less restrictive of the person's rights and freedom of action"

As a reminder, the principles are outlined in Table 4.1 (see Chapter 1 for a full discussion of the MCA, 2005, and the equivalent Scottish and Northern Irish legislation).

In addition, an individual does not have the capacity to make a decision if they are unable to satisfy any one of the four conditions in the 'incapacity test'; Section 3 of the MCA (2005) provides the test that should be used. A person is unable to make a decision for himself if he is unable:

(a) To understand the information relevant to the decision

(b) To retain that information

(c) To use or weigh that information as part of the process of making the decision, or

(d) To communicate his decision (whether by talking, using sign language or any other means).

The historical assumption that people living with dementia are unable to participate in making decisions about their health and care has long been challenged (Dewing, 2007b, 2008; Dresser, 1995; Dworkin, 1993; Jaworska, 1999). There are now also multiple sources of evidence which demonstrate that people living with dementia can reliably report on their values and preferences in relation to their care, wellbeing, and quality of life, even in moderate and late stage dementia (Boyle, 2014; Feinberg, 2002; Whitlatch, Feinberg, & Tucke, 2005).

Professionals should not be unduly influenced by what Judge Ryder has termed as the "protection imperative" (the perceived need to protect a vulnerable adult) (Oldham MBC v GW and PW [2007] EWHC 136 (Fam), 2007) arguing that "The person need only comprehend and weigh the salient details relevant to the decision and not all the peripheral detail. Moreover, different individuals may give different weight to different factors" (LBL v RYJ, 2010 paras 24,58). "[T]here is a risk that all professionals involved with treating and helping that person … may feel drawn towards an outcome that is more protective of the adult and thus… fail to carry out an assessment of capacity that is detached and objective."("CC v. KK and STCC," 2012).

Practical Tip

Wherever possible it is important to support people to use remaining capacity and extant abilities by choosing suitable times, tools and environments to facilitate their decision-making ability – remember to use your skills to help them use what they have.

Finally in this section, it would be unforgivable to explore the MCA in extended care settings without mentioning The Deprivation of Liberty Safeguards (SCIE, 2007) (reviewed by the Law Commission and presented to the Government in March 2017 as the Liberty Protection Safeguards – currently awaiting implementation; see http://www.lawcom.gov.uk/project/mental-capacity-and-deprivation-of-liberty/ for further information).

DoLS were appended to the MCA (2005) as a response to the HL v UK [2004] 'Bournewood' case, where it became clear that a significant number of people were being detained illegally by health and social care providers for care and treatment without valid consent, due to a gap in the legislation in breach of the European Convention Human Rights (ECHR) (1998) *Article 5* 'Right to liberty'.

Following the Bournewood judgement it became clear that a legal framework was required to ensure that the human rights of incapacitous individuals were upheld, whilst also enabling the application of the MCA to ensure that necessary and appropriate care and treatment could be delivered safely in a person's best interests. The case law shaped the way that DoLS legislation was implemented and how a deprivation of liberty was interpreted, until the crucial 'Cheshire West case' (P v Cheshire West & Chester Council, 2014) when Baroness Hale highlighted what she termed as the 'acid test'. The 'acid test' (is the individual free to leave, and are they under complete supervision and control) was always the legal stance, but this ruling changed the application of the process virtually overnight.

Case study 1 Deprivation of Liberty assessment

As 70% of people in care homes are living with dementia, it seems appropriate to review the basics of dementia and reflect on its potential impact on an individual's decision-making capacity. This case study relates to a real situation, and highlights some of the major and minor decisions that people are faced with.

Case study 1

P is a 96-year-old farmer who has been living in a nursing home for the past 13 years. He was initially detained under the Mental Health Act (1983) when he was admitted to an acute mental health facility from home following a period of self-neglect which resulted in multiple arterial leg ulcers and malnutrition. Following a relatively short period in the hospital ward P was transferred to the nursing home where he now resides. The original transfer and detention was undertaken on an 'informal' basis without P's consent. P was in his room when I visited (to undertake a DoLS assessment) and he told me to 'F*** off' as he was watching his favourite television programme. The nurse obviously had a good rapport with P and suggested that he might like to take time out from the television, which he did reluctantly.

P has a diagnosis of vascular dementia and is able to mobilize with a stick. The nurse highlights that he requires assistance unless he wants to get into bed during the day when he manages 'just fine on his own'. Although P appears quite physically frail he is very strong and sometimes physically declines and resists personal care. This is highlighted as an issue due to occasional double incontinence; this is dealt with using chemical restraint. Family members are regularly involved in and supportive of P's care so there is no need for an Independent Mental Capacity Advocate (IMCA) to be appointed.

It may be useful to reflect on:

- Whether you believe the appointment time and/or environment had, (or could have) any impact on P's ability to make a decision about his place of residence

- P is clearly able to demonstrate his likes and dislikes. We chatted about what he likes to do and whether he was happy in the care home. P said that he was as happy as could be expected under the circumstances, he had his 'easy' chair from home which he liked and would sit in most of the day, and had a paper every morning; he had a nice window although he complained of not actually being outside enough. P seemed to think that he had no choice. P then asked who

I was and started to get agitated and commenced shouting. His nurse came and sat quietly with P and I withdrew to consider the documentation.

- Whether you believe P has the capacity to make decisions about personal care
- Whether P does have a choice regarding his accommodation
- Anything else that you noticed
- The tools, expertise or advice you could offer to P and/or his care staff that could have a positive impact on his life and care.

The use of assessment forms can create a positive structure for MCA assessments (and demonstrate the importance of documentation throughout the process both for the individual and for the practitioner). A more fluid approach, however, may support relationship building and create a more enabling and supportive atmosphere for the individual to make their own decisions.

Reflections on case study 1

- It may be that both the appointment time and environment had an impact on P's ability to make a decision about his place of residence but in very different ways. As his personal space, the environment potentially had a positive impact on P with his personal belongings around him; it was calm, confidential and quiet. However, the time of the appointment clearly interfered with a favourite TV programme and this could have easily been avoided.

Practical Tip

It is worth being mindful as a visiting professional that care home staff will often put themselves and their residents out to work around your busy diary. Whilst this appears kind and accommodating you don't always get the best out of the person that you are visiting.

- Whether P has the capacity to make decisions about personal care is tricky because that assessment can only be made in the moment that he requires personal care. It may be worth considering (1) who is the personal care for? This might seem like a ridiculous question but is the smell causing issues for other residents or distress and discomfort for P? (2) Does P understand the consequences of not having personal care (for his skin health, for example)?(3) Are nurses/care staff imposing their own hygiene standards and routines on P who may have historically only washed or bathed weekly?

- It appears that P actually has no choice regarding his accommodation.

- P reported that he would like to be outside more. Encouraging him to be outside and use his skills in the garden could have a positive impact on his daily life. P also said that he was as happy as could be expected, so offering him the opportunity for person-centred useful occupation of his time might enhance his life and care and reduce his episodes of agitation.

Care partners

At home, care partners (relatives and friends) support their loved ones to communicate their values and needs. Moving into a care home can change this relationship and support, largely because the care partner is no longer constantly available due to time or geographical constraints. Care partners play an essential role in helping care staff to find out what matters to care home residents and shaping person-centred care.

Although care partner involvement is important, it should be sought to accompany information from the person living with dementia and not to supersede it. Regardless of the other parties involved, the person living with the cognitive impairment must at least be given the opportunity to choose to participate in the decision-making process (Miller, Whitlatch, & Lyons, 2014).

In practice, many care settings (not just care homes) rely upon family members to make decisions for people living with dementia, regardless of legal, medical, or ethical processes (Miller et al., 2014). It is also always important to check if people have made any advanced decision prior to commencing an assessment and to remember that care partners may have a Lasting Power of Attorney (LPA) for personal welfare and/or property and affairs. And this arrangement has legal standing if it is registered (further information is available at http://www.legislation.gov.uk/ukpga/2005/9/part/1/crossheading/

lasting-powers-of-attorney). Even if it is not registered it may be important to the person in question and as such is important to consider.

Case study 2 The Mental Capacity Assessment

Q is a musically gifted and highly-educated gentleman who suffered a traumatic brain injury as a result of a road traffic accident 15 years ago. He received intensive physiotherapy, psychological support, speech and language and occupational therapies for two years until the medical team predicted that little or no further improvements could be made. At this point he was transferred to an extended care environment. Q speaks very rapidly and can be difficult to understand until one has become attuned to his speech, although he has strong verbal communication skills and is easily understood by those who know him well. He remembers names and is somewhat uninhibited following his accident which can put him at risk. Q regularly says that he would like to go home.

Q has a self-contained flat within the care home where he lives 'alone' and has 24-hour care. Q's care plans highlight that he has limited ability to recognize and manage risk, although Q is clear that he had been prone to risk-taking prior to his accident; in fact, he says that his accident was as a result of his risk-taking behaviour. Q is free to come and go as he pleases – under the constant supervision of his carer – and chooses his own activities such as bowling, the cinema, concerts and going to the pub. He also enjoys gaming and watching movies at home. Q is independent with regard to his activities of daily living and has no medical or nursing needs identified.

In order to assess Q's capacity to choose his place of residence one must systematically employ the five key principles of the MCA (2005) framework. It is useful to identify a specific question such as "Do you want to continue to live at this care home?" because the Act focuses on the particular matter at the specified time, not on any theoretical ability to make decisions generally. It may be more difficult than you think to identify the right question!

Undertaking this assessment takes professional skill and judgement in addition to objectivity. The more experience you gain in undertaking assessments or supporting assessments the more these skills will be enhanced.

The following questions will support you to reflect on the case with the five key principles in mind:

Principle 1: Presumption of capacity Would you look at Q's records or have extended discussions with care staff prior to meeting Q? Would this influence your ability to assume Q's full capacity?

Principle 2: Maximizing involvement Where would you undertake Q's assessment? How would you decide the time of the assessment? What skills would you employ to ensure that you maximized Q's involvement in the decision?

Principle 3: Unwise decisions Could you support Q to make what you might consider an unwise decision, for example, if he wishes to return to home where he may not be safe? How does supporting an unwise decision that puts a service user in danger conflict with your professional duty of care? How does it make you feel?

Principle 4: Best interests If Q was assessed as lacking capacity, what are your thoughts about best interest considerations? Who would you involve? What would be your primary goals?

Principle 5: Less restriction How could Q's care be provided in a way that "is less restrictive of the person's rights and freedom of action" (Mental Capacity Act s1 (6))?

Taking the time to reflect on this case may give you the opportunity to explore your own thoughts and feelings about more than this specific case. Do you feel conflicted about facilitating 'unwise' decisions? Are you comfortable about performing MCA assessments? There are many practitioners from all healthcare professions (including doctors) who will pass on this key responsibility if they can. However, as an SLT, who is vital to this process for many people living with cognitive impairment, this may not be so easy to do.

Reflections on case study 2

• **Principle 1: Presumption of capacity**

It can be useful to meet the person prior to exploring the care plans and risk assessment paperwork because it provides the opportunity to decide if an assessment is actually required. This can be contentious but it is difficult to presume capacity when all the documentation suggests that it is lacking. On what grounds is the mental capacity assessment being undertaken? Be clear that there is sufficient evidence that Q may lack capacity otherwise this may constitute a breach of Principle 1.

- **Principle 2: Maximizing involvement**

In an ideal world Q's assessment would take place at the time and place of his choosing (if he has the ability to choose). There will be instances when the person is unable to communicate where or when they want their assessment, and using a consultee and/or the person who knows them best may be helpful. For instance, a person's own home or a quiet room rather than behind a curtain in a busy ward, not at lunchtime or clashing with a favourite TV programme (as in case study 1); these small, simple things can make a big difference. It is also worth remembering that a Mini Mental State Examination (MMSE) score does not reflect an individual's ability to make decisions. The skills you employ to ensure that you maximize Q's involvement in the decision will largely depend on your assessment of Q and how best to communicate with him.

- **Principle 3: Unwise decisions**

Supporting someone to make what you might consider an unwise decision is difficult. But if it is perceived that an individual understands the consequence of that decision there is a duty to support them, however uncomfortable that might make you feel. Supporting an unwise decision which puts a service user in potential danger conflicts with our professional duty of care and only you know how that makes you feel.

- **Principle 4: Best interests**

Professionals may use 'best interests' as a justification for doing something that *they* think is in the person's best interest. Best interest considerations should always be based on what that person would perceive to be in their own best interest to our knowledge and that is why it is so important to involve them and their family and friends in those decisions.

- **Principle 5: Less restriction**

Care that is provided in a way that is "less restrictive of the person's rights and freedom of action" is as much about the person's rights as their physical environment, and this may be overlooked. Therefore, following the other four principles and always putting Q at the centre of his care, respecting his rights and wishes are as important as where or how physical restrictions are implemented.

Process consent and the MCA

Recognition of the need to directly involve people living with cognitive and communication impairments in decisions that affect their health and care is increasing. The MCA strengthens the case for their active inclusion for as long as possible, emphasized by the first principle – the presumption of capacity unless there is evidence to the contrary. Some impairments or disturbances are permanent or may be degenerative. In other instances, capacity will fluctuate or fully return. Thus, the Act makes it clear that a lack of capacity cannot be assumed or established merely by reference to a person's age, appearance or behaviour. The United Nations Convention on the Rights of People with Disabilities (United Nations, 2006) furthers the argument that, regardless of disability, people are entitled to be regarded and treated as equals. Recognition of ongoing emotional, relational, aesthetic and spiritual abilities is essential to maintaining meaningful social inclusion for people living with dementia.

Ongoing process consent is a method of seeking consent from people living with dementia and other cognitive difficulties. In this model consent is continually sought and renegotiated (Dewing, 2007a; Gelling & Munn-Giddings, 2011). Process consent is not (as some people have suggested) an excuse to 'dodge the MCA' but is actually a useful tool to facilitate decision-making participation whilst respecting the legislative framework and protecting the person and those that fulfil caring roles. Using this method requires a high level of skill and self-awareness on the part of the practitioner and builds on work to progress inclusion, empowerment and choice for people living with dementia (e.g., Bartlett & O'Connor, 2010; Hubbard, Downs, & Tester, 2003; Martin & Younger, 2000)

Process consent (Dewing, 2007a, 2008) involves a five stage model (see Table 4.2) that aims to offer people living with dementia and limited or fluctuating capacity, the opportunity to be involved and included in decisions that may previously not have been considered possible. It relies on information being tailored to people's individual needs. As such it may resonate with SLTs as 'normal practice'; using their core communication skills to facilitate and reveal capacity in the person they are working with.

Table 4.2 The Process Consent Method (Dewing, 2008).

One: Background and preparation Firstly, engage with gatekeepers (family or professional) to confirm access to the person living with dementia. It is stressed that this is not proxy consent and you should be transparent about negotiations. This process enables care partners authorized by the person living with dementia to be instrumental in the process. A basic biography of the person is required including indications and usual levels of wellbeing. This may include a description of facial expressions or behaviours generally exhibited for different levels of wellbeing.
Two: Establishing the basis for consent Explore existing capacity assessments and/or opinions, recognizing that capacity is time- and decision-specific. Poor MMSE scores do not equate to a loss of capacity but enable you to identify more creative and sensitive methods tailored to include the individual. If the individual does not have capacity to consent to participate in the decision, you should establish to what extent the person can make their own choices, and how they feel about the decision in question. Consent established in this way relies on a more holistic perspective of the person and not on the conventional cognitive emphasis on understanding, retaining and weighing of information. It is important to recognize that this is not informed consent and must be revisited continuously, sensitive to any conversation or behaviour that might indicate a psycho-therapeutic need.
Three: Initial consent Consent now becomes entirely specific to the individual. You assess the individual's communication needs and abilities and provide information tailored in such a way that it is meaningful to that person and is modified to their strengths and residual abilities.
Four: On going consent monitoring Consent must be revisited and re-established on, and within, every element of the decision. Ongoing consent may be assessed against the initial consent, for consistency, and transparency gained through validation from a care partner or key worker. This encourages independent verification of the person's wellbeing.
Five: Feedback and support If feedback to care partners, staff and/or supervisors is considered necessary regarding concerns around an individual's wellbeing then confidentiality needs to be carefully considered. Feedback should always be agreed with the person living with dementia beforehand, if possible.

The value of the SLT in care home decision making

When one reflects on the figures discussed above, detailing the number of people living with dementia in care homes and the lack of training offered to most care staff, it is unsurprising that they need help and support from visiting professionals. Yet, despite the fact that most people living with dementia will develop language or communication difficulties at some point in their dementia trajectory SLTs are infrequently called on for their expertise in communication facilitation.

Whilst people in care homes are regularly referred to SLT, this is almost always for advice on swallowing and not for support around language or communication needs. As a Registered Nurse and Best Interest Assessor this is an absolute travesty in my opinion, for both people living with dementia and for their care staff and partners. SLTs can change the lived experience of people in care homes with minimal input by sharing their expertise with care staff and teaching them to use tools to support people to communicate. The SLT can support staff to support people to participate in daily activities and decisions, improve their quality of life and reduce distress-related behaviours – in short, taking back some control of their care.

The care home population is complex, and needs (and deserves) the support of the entire multidisciplinary team. I have met with care staff who have printed pictures from the internet in an effort to support an aphasic stroke survivor. I have seen staff sit for hours trying to calm a person living with dementia, who shouts constantly. In my experience, care home staff are ready and willing to learn any skills that you can offer and would gratefully accept your support with MCA assessments and other communication-related challenges that they face.

When one considers the MCA and the fact that the ability to communicate a decision features so highly, one would imagine that health and social care commissioners would be employing additional SLTs to support people with decision making to ensure that they comply with the law. Yet nothing appears to have changed, despite the MCA (2005) and subsequently the Care Act (2012). This is undoubtedly a commissioning issue and cannot be resolved until SLT's communication skills receive the recognition they deserve. Yet, raising the profile of SLTs in care homes by supporting staff, with hints and tips to help them communicate better, would start to have an impact in ensuring that your service is high on the commissioning agenda. Ultimately raising the profile of the profession with commissioners has the potential to increase staffing resources.

So, next time you do a swallow assessment with a person living with dementia, comment on the individual's communication as well. Ask about how they manage and if they need support. Mention its relevance to decision making. This will remind the team of the breadth of your role. Perhaps you could ask for a list of all the people in the care home who would benefit from communication assessment input. Can you do an audit or a project to assess the need and the impact at this care home? Perhaps pilot staff training and assess the impact? Use student SLTs creatively?

Managers and commissioners should be encouraged to use audit results and outcomes data demonstrating the need and the impact of involving SLTs in communication support in care homes. Focusing on the potential positive outcomes can be useful, such as: happier residents and staff, less distressed behaviours, less paperwork, less staff turnover, reduced recruitment budget. Equally focusing on risks may also be useful: how many capacity assessments could have benefited from the involvement of an SLT? Is there a risk register in your Trust where this could be flagged? Other health or care professionals can support this process too. Asking other professionals to refer to you or to ask for advice on communication can demonstrate need.

Discussion

Imagine moving to a foreign country. You don't really want to go but your family will be going with you. You don't know the language or the area and the satnav keeps sending you in the wrong direction. You try to learn the language and when people speak slowly and clearly you can understand elements of what they are trying to explain. Pictures or maps sometimes help too, and you start to get by quite nicely. Then one day, for no apparent reason, you find yourself in a different land where the landscape is completely alien. Each way that you turn everything looks the same and this time your family is not here. People are kind but you don't understand them and they don't understand you.

- How do you feel?

- What do you need to make it different or acceptable to you?

- How can you express your feelings if no-one understands your language?

- Are you scared or do you feel liberated?

- Are you excited at the prospect of engaging in a new adventure or lonely and looking for a way back?

This reflects a conversation that I had with a lovely older lady living with early dementia in a care home. She explained so brilliantly how her mixed dementia made her feel. She was kind and sweet and quiet, and became quieter and quieter. She could speak but it 'came out wrong' and she was embarrassed. She loved to have her hand held. Many older people that I have cared for miss touch. This is sometimes described as 'skin hunger'. It is so easily rectified with a kind hand.

The care home supported her and she was happy most of the time. She had family visitors every week – sometimes 3-4 times. Later, she would forget that she had visitors moments after they had left and sometimes she had no idea who they were, except that they were familiar and she liked them. Her terrible frustration rarely erupted in 'challenging behaviour' (a label that is actually a call for help). This sweet old lady was my grandmother.

SLTs have the skills to act as translators in this foreign land of dementia, and to give other health and care staff basic instruction to help them do the same. They can help people to feel included and important and listened to.

Summary

This chapter focused on people living with dementia and other cognitive impairments in care homes and the people, practitioners and services that support them. The strengths and limitations of the health and care services have been discussed and used to highlight where SLTs may be able to use their professional knowledge and skills to influence the care of individuals; from simple training and tools to entire systems.

Influencing commissioners to ensure that this vulnerable population has access to specialist SLT knowledge and skills is key. Working with this client group is complex. And although this complexity may be recognized, the role of the SLT in supporting people who may lack capacity in these settings may not yet be adequately valued. This seems an important step to ensuring true multidisciplinary support in mental capacity assessments within the care home setting.

Relevant statutes

2014 Care Act

2007 Mental Health Act

2005 Mental Capacity Act

1983 Mental Health Act

Useful documents and websites

- 39 Essex Chambers, Mental Capacity Law http://www.39essex.com/resources-and-training/mental-capacity-law/
- Association of Directors of Adult Social Services (2015) Deprivation of Liberty Safeguards Form 3 Combined Age, Mental Capacity, No Refusals and Best Interests http://www.adass.org.uk/mental-health-Drugs-and-Alcohol/key-documents/New-DoLS-Forms/
- Centre for Workforce Intelligence (2012). Discussion document. Shape of the Medical Workforce: Starting the debate on the future consultant workforce
- European Convention Human Rights (1998) https://www.liberty-human-rights.org.uk/human-rights/what-are-human-rights/human-rights-act/article-5-right-liberty
- Department of Health (2014) Positive and Proactive Care: Reducing the need for restrictive interventions. London: DH
- Ministry of Justice (2008) Mental Capacity Act 2005 Deprivation of Liberty Safeguards code of practice to supplement the main MCA 2005 code of practice. London: TSO
- NHS Information Centre (2012). Report. NHS Workforce: Summary of staff in the NHS: Results from September 2011 census
- Office of the Public Guardian https://www.gov.uk/government/organisations/office-of-the-public-guardian
- Select Committee on the Mental Capacity Act 2005 Report: post-legislative scrutiny http://www.publications.parliament.uk/pa/ld201314/ldselect/ldmentalcap/139/13902.htm
- Skills for Care (2011). Report. The Size and Structure of the Adult Social Care Sector and Workforce in England, 2011

References

Bartlett, R. & O'Connor, D. (2010). *Broadening the Dementia Debate: Towards Social Citizenship*. London: Policy Press.

Boyle, G. (2014). Recognising the agency of people with dementia. *Disability & Society, 29*(7), 1130-1144.1. doi:10.1080/09687599.2014.910108

Bunn, F., Burn, A.-M., Goodman, C., Rait, G., Norton, S., Robinson, L., . . . Brayne, C. (2014). Comorbidity and dementia: A scoping review of the literature. *BMC Medicine, 12*(1), 1.

CC v. KK and STCC, No. 2136 (EWHC 2012).

Care Act 2014, http://www.legislation.gov.uk/ukpga/2014/23/contents/enacted (2014).

Clarke, A.M., Davey, M.F., & Horner, B.J. (2004). Communication and decision making among residents with dementia. *Geriaction, 22*(3), 17-24.

Commission on Residential Care. (2014). *A Vision for Care Fit for the 21st Century.* London: Demos.

Department for Constitutional Affairs. (2007). *Mental Capacity Act 2005 Code of Practice.* London: The Stationery Office.

Dewing, J. (2007). Participatory research: A method for process consent with persons who have dementia. *Dementia, 6*(1), 11-25.

Dewing, J. (2008). Process consent and research with older persons living with dementia. *Research Ethics Review, 4*(2), 59-64.

Dresser, R. (1995). Dworkin on dementia: Elegant theory, questionable policy. *Hastings Centre Report, 25*(6), 32-38. doi:10.2307/3527839

Dworkin, R.M. (1993). *Life's Dominion: An Argument about Abortion, Euthanasia, and Individual Freedom.* New York: Vintage Books.

Feinberg, L.F. & Whitlatch, J. (2002). Decision-making for persons with cognitive impairment and their family caregivers. *American Journal of Alzheimer's Disease and Other Dementias, 17*(4), 237-244.

Gelling, L. & Munn-Giddings, C. (2011). Ethical review of action research: The challenges for researchers and research ethics committees. *Research Ethics, 7*(3), 100-106.

Gladman, J.R. & Bowman, C.E. (2012). *Quality of Care and the Quality of Life in Care Homes.* Oxford: Oxford University Press.

Goodman, C., Amador, S., Elmore, N., Machen, I., & Mathie, E. (2013). Preferences and priorities for ongoing and end-of-life care: A qualitative study of older people with dementia resident in care homes. *International Journal of Nursing Studies, 50*(12), 1639-1647.

Handley, M., Bunn, F., & Goodman, C. (2017). Dementia-friendly interventions to improve the care of people living with dementia admitted to hospitals: A realist review. *BMJ Open, 7*(7), e015257.

Hubbard, G., Downs, M.G., & Tester, S. (2003). Including older people with dementia in research: Challenges and strategies. *Aging and Mental Health, 7*(5), 351-362.

Jaworska, A. (1999). Respecting the margins of agency: Alzheimer's patients and the capacity to value. *Philosophy & Public Affairs, 28*(2), 105-138. doi:10.1111/j.1088-4963.1999.00105.x

Law Commission, The (1991). *Mentally Incapacitated Adults and Decision-making: An Overview.* London: HM Stationery Office.

LBL v RYJ No. 2664 (Fam) (EWHC 2010).

Martin, G.W. & Younger, D. (2000). Anti oppressive practice: A route to the empowerment of people with dementia through communication and choice. *Psychiatric Mental Health Nursing*, 7(1), 59-67.

Matthews, F.E., Arthur, A., Barnes, L.E., Bond, J., Jagger, C., Robinson, L., & Brayne, C. (2013). A two-decade comparison of prevalence of dementia in individuals aged 65 years and older from three geographical areas of England: Results of the Cognitive Function and Ageing Study I and II. *The Lancet*, 382(9902), 1405-1412.

Miller, L.M., Whitlatch, C.J., & Lyons, K.S. (2014). Shared decision-making in dementia: A review of patient and family carer involvement. *Dementia*, 15, 1141-1157. doi:10.1177/1471301214555542

Oldham MBC v GW and PW, No. 136 (Fam) (EWHC 2007).

P v Cheshire West & Chester Council (2014).

Prince, M., Knapp, M., Guerchet, M., McCrone, P., Prina, M., Comas-Herrera, A., . . . King, D. (2014). *Dementia UK: Update*. London: Alzheimer's Society.

Quality Care Commission. (2014). *Cracks in the Pathway*. London: CQC.

United Nations. (2006). *Convention on the Rights of Persons with Disabilities (CRPD)*. New York: United Nations.

Whitlatch, C.J., Feinberg, L.F., & Tucke, S.S. (2005). Measuring the values and preferences for everyday care of persons with cognitive impairment and their family caregivers. *Gerontologist*, 45(3), 370-380.

5 Communication skills training to support decision making

Anna Volkmer

Introduction

For some time now speech and language therapists (SLTs) have included communication training in their repertoire of therapeutic interventions. The research evidence in this area demonstrates that training parents can improve their interactions with their children (Allen & Marshall, 2015), training nursing staff and healthcare professionals can improve their interactions with people with dementia (Eggenberger, Heimeri, & Bennett, 2012), and training family members can improve conversations with loved ones with post-stroke aphasia (Simmons-Mackie, Savage, & Worrall, 2014). The research evidence demonstrating that SLTs can train healthcare professionals or family members to improve interactions with people with dementia, traumatic brain injury and other mental health conditions is fairly widely accepted. This evidence also suggests that SLTs should have a direct role in supporting and training people (professionals and anyone else involved in decision making) to communicate better with individuals (with communication difficulties) who may lack decision-making capacity.

Communication training of this kind may take different forms: it may be delivered to a group using a generic approach, or delivered on an individual basis, developed to the specific needs of the people involved. Communication training may include the person with the communication difficulty, or may be delivered only to the communication partner or partners. Communication training may be didactic – a one-off lecture – or may include tasks whereby the participants have the opportunity to practise what they are learning. Some of these approaches are considered more effective, others more practical and time efficient, and may be used for different reasons in different settings.

To support you in planning and developing communication skills training, the following discussion provides an overview of different approaches to communication skills training and how these may be applied to support people who may lack decision-making capacity. The evidence in the area of communication skills training is presented and the practical components subsequently summarized. This chapter is distinct from Chapter 6 in this book; this chapter focuses on verbal interactions and the use of strategies, whilst the other focuses on training others to use accessible written information. In short, both these chapters may be useful to you when developing your training materials. Their content is different but complementary. These ideas may be used to construct training sessions for staff in care facilities such as those described in Chapter 4, or in multidisciplinary training such as described in Chapter 2.

Who are we training?

The draft NICE guidelines for decision making and mental capacity that went out for public consultation early in 2018 made a number of recommendations with regard to communication skills training firstly advocating that:

> "responsible bodies should ensure all practitioners undergo training to help them to apply the Mental Capacity Act 2005 and its Code of Practice"

and that this should include "required communication skills" and, secondly, that specific communication skills training is required as distinct from other types of training in relation to decision making and mental capacity. (Of note these guidelines are a draft and may not remain the same in the final version due for publication at time of writing in October 2018).

These recommendations emphasize the value of communication skills training. They suggest both that health and social care professionals require this training be provided by the organization they work with and that specific communication skills training is required as distinct from other types of training in relation to decision making and mental capacity.

The RCSLT is very clear on its position about the role of the SLT in training. It states that, "The RCSLT consider that all professionals involved in the capacity assessment including advocates, should receive mandatory training from a

SLT to ensure that they are able to understand and use the most appropriate mode and level of communication with the individual" (RCSLT, 2014, p. 6).

The research literature also highlights the area of need at the individual level. "89% of nursing staff respondents identified working with service users with dementia as very or quite challenging, with a particular training need being around communication. Ineffective communication risks misunderstanding, failure to address needs, disappointment or distress" (Allwood et al., 2017, p. 213). Ultimately, misunderstandings can also mean that people are not given the right to participate in decisions about their own care. Providing people with the tools (through training) to reduce these barriers and improve accessibility to decision making is an important role for SLTs.

Communication skills training for groups of professionals

What do people want and need from your training? Before you start planning your actual training, you need to consider the broader issues. What is driving the provision of this training? Who is going to attend the training? What are you going to do and how? How will you make sure this has a lasting impact for attendees, those they work with, and those who organized the training? Chapter 8 in this book sets out an in-depth discussion around evaluation and its relevance to this type of training. It would be worth reading that chapter before you progress much further in planning your actual training session.

The Medical Research Council (MRC) provides guidance on how complex

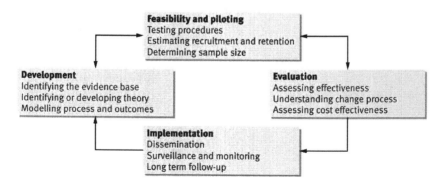

Figure 5.1 Development and evaluation process for complex interventions (based on Craig et al., 2008).

interventions should be measured and evaluated (Craig, 2008). Communication skills training can be considered a complex intervention. The MRC explains that there is a process to developing, piloting, evaluating and implementing these types of interventions. Figure 5.1 summarizes the key components of this cycle. It is not feasible to propose that clinicians approach the development of a training programme in this way unless they are considering a formal research project. Nevertheless, it is worth considering the model as a good practice structure for developing services and translating this to the clinical setting. Figure 5.2 proposes how this type of model may be used to plan communication skills training in a more clinical setting.

Having considered the stages required in planning an intervention this chapter will then focus predominantly on the development stage of the communication skills training. The current research evidence in the area of

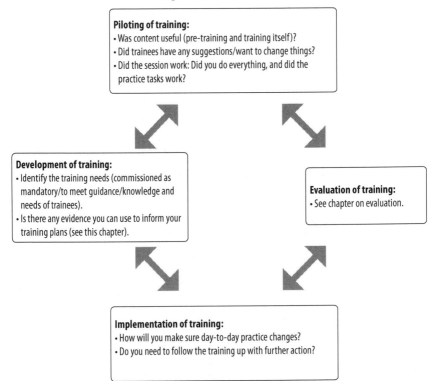

Figure 5.2 Modifying the development and evaluation process for a clinical communication skills training programme.

communication skills training relevant to decision making and mental capacity is presented and specific activities in relation to communication skills training are discussed.

Development of training: Training needs

Has the training you are doing been commissioned to meet a mandatory requirement, or a guideline? In this case, will the training need to be delivered to a large number of people repeatedly over a number of years? And should the same content be presented in an identical method at each training session? Should there be a need for this type of consistency then you may wish to explore the medium of delivery. You can consider an online training video or lecture, or a standardized PowerPoint lecture. The content of this type of training can be planned in advance and delivered in exactly the same way each time.

Should the training be driven by the needs of the attendees then you may choose to adopt a more dynamic approach and consider asking what they would like you to deliver in the training. It can be helpful to share what people have identified in advance at the training session. People find it reassuring and may even find suggestions more believable when their peers (who are hopefully using these strategies) suggest them. Lanzi and colleagues (2017) suggest that "Training begins by establishing rapport with caregivers by first asking questions about challenges in caring for their family member. This involves listening to their concerns, and then offering suggestions and support" (Lanzi, Burshnic, & Bourgeouis, 2017, p. 371). In achieving something similar you may wish to visit staff you are planning to train to ask them in person what they would like. For example, perhaps they are colleagues and you could ask about a particular service user they may wish to discuss. Using cases can contextualize the training to make it relevant. Inviting them to bring their own cases for problem solving or discussion may be a good way to deal with real problems, and may ensure attendees carry over strategies into a real-life situation. If they are unable to discuss a real service user, you might consider using vignettes or case studies to prompt problem-solving discussions, or focus on practice tasks/role plays.

Development of training:
Evidence to inform your training plans

There are numerous examples of the effectiveness of communication skills training in the research literature. As with all examples from the research literature, though, it is worth considering the rigour of the study and the relevance to the people you are working with. This may include considering when it was written, what research has been done in the area since then and, ideally, searching for a systematic review that brings together and compares the research for you. The following discussion considers some evidence from both the dementia and the aphasia literature.

Communication training from dementia and aphasia: The evidence

FOCUSED is a communication skills training programme designed for nursing staff working with people with Alzheimer's disease by Ripich (1994). The authors demonstrated that 17 nursing assistants who were trained using the FOCUSED programme showed increased control over social interaction and improved satisfaction in social interaction following the intervention (Ripich, Ziol, & Lee, 1998).

FOCUSED sessions typically run for one or two hours per week over four to eight weeks and are presented by an SLT using the FOCUSED programme. The programme includes discussion questions, videotaped vignettes, role-play activities, a caregiver's guide and prompt card. This is a seven-step programme teaching specific conversation skills under the following headings:

Face: Face the person, call his name, touch him, gain and maintain eye contact.

Orient: Orient the person to the topic by repeating key words several times, repeat and rephrase sentences, use nouns and specific names.

Continue: Continue the same topic of conversation for as long as possible, restate the topic throughout the conversation, indicate to the person when you are introducing a new topic.

Un-stick: Help the person become 'unstuck' when he or she uses a word incorrectly by suggesting the intended word, repeat the sentence the person said using the correct word, ask "Do you mean...?"

Structured: Structure your questions so the person will be able to recognize and repeat a response, provide two simple choices at a time, use yes/no questions.

Exchange: Keep up the normal exchange of ideas used in everyday conversation, keep conversations going with comments such as, "Oh how nice", or "That's great", do not ask test questions, give the person clues as to how to answer your questions.

Direct: Keep sentences short, simple and direct, put the subject of the sentences first, use and repeat nouns (names) rather than pronouns (he, she, it), use hand signals, pictures and facial expressions.

Ripich et al. (1998) refined the training to meet the needs of caregivers. In later studies, they describe training 19 caregivers (family members and spouses) of people with mid-stage Alzheimer's disease using the FOCUSED programme and compared this group to a control group of family members and carers who received no input. Results showed that FOCUSED group participants rated communication 'hassles' as having decreased over time, whilst knowledge about Alzheimer's disease increased. This was reviewed 12 months after the training, and improvements were maintained. In short, understanding communication breakdown in Alzheimer's' disease and learning how to cope with these results reduced the care burden for relatives of people with dementia. The authors hypothesize that caregivers require time to practise and integrate information and strategies before they can have an impact on conversation. They suggest that this development in the successful implementation of strategies also supports their ongoing use and therefore maintenance of results at 12 months. It is important to note, however, that many of the strategies used in this programme are those that have been found not to be useful in other research which surveyed the perceived usefulness of a series of strategies by caregivers and family members (Small & Gutman, 2002). This probably highlights the importance of individualized approaches even when planning a group intervention.

Ripich and colleagues (1999) continued their research into the use of the FOCUSED programme with 32 caregivers of people with dementia. The caregivers attended training over four-weekly, one-hour sessions. The researchers were able to demonstrate specific improvements in the types of questions used by carers, particularly the increased use of closed questions and the consequent increase in successful responses from the person they cared for. They also introduced booster groups, which did not really result in any increase in maintenance of skills when compared with those who did not attend booster groups. They suggest that future maintenance might be best enhanced though more personally relevant support. This echoes some of the previous comments highlighted by Small and Gutman (2002).

Since then numerous communication training approaches for carers working with people with dementia have been reported in the research literature. Consequently, Eggenberger et al. (2013) published a systematic literature review of these studies that aimed to "evaluate interventions that have been designed to enhance communication or interaction in dementia care in any setting". The review found 12 trials, seven of which were randomized controlled trials in nursing homes and domestic settings. In care home settings training usually started with an in-service training (a lecture of talk) in small groups. Individual training was more common in people's homes. Training varied in duration and intensity from between 2 two-hour sessions to 13 one-hour sessions, or 2 eight-hour sessions with additional practical training tasks, including feedback for observed interactions. Tasks described included:

- Small group discussions on frustration and personal experiences
- Brainstorming sessions on successful and unsuccessful communication
- Role-play
- Problem-based learning such as case discussions of example or real vignettes
- Reflecting situations from daily care routine
- Discussion tasks including taking the perspective of people with dementia in vignettes and agreeing written behaviour management plans
- Using video to present and illustrate examples in the educational component of the training
- Using audio and video to analyze communication breakdown and successful use of strategies
- Providing workbooks, handouts, booklets, memory books, prompt cards with strategies, references for further reading.

The content of all the 12 communication skills training trials is summarized by Eggenberger et al. (2013). Table 5.1 provides their summary of the verbal, nonverbal and emotional skills and the knowledge about communication issues that were delivered across the studies.

Table 5.1 Content of communication skills training in dementia care (Eggenberger et al., 2013; Table 4).

Content of communication skills training in dementia care
Verbal skills
Before physical care
Announce single activities
Use one-step instructions, no usage of multiple instructions
Delay physical assistance after verbal prompt
At an early stage of illness trajectory
Avoid arguing, accept different perceptions of time and reality
Use of yes/no and choice questions versus open-ended questions
Suggest words when person is struggling for a specific word
At a moderate to late stage of illness trajectory
Use names and nouns
Use the person's name
Use simple sentences
Repeat and rephrase sentences
General skills
Use positive and biographical statements
Identify personal communication styles and preferences
Identify and do not use elder speak (diminutives, pronoun substitutions)
Slow down
Nonverbal and emotional skills
Recognize unusual communicative attempts
Recognize micro-behavioural changes (eye movement, lifting the corner of the mouth, tears, etc.) as attempts to communicate
View behaviour that challenges as an attempt to communicate unmet needs
Reflect your own nonverbal behaviour
Make eye contact
Give enough time
Avoid high-pitch voice
Listen actively
Recognize and answer to emotions
Notice and validate person with dementia's effects
Use emotional tone
Show empathy
Knowledge on communication issues
Know about changes in communication with older people in general (hearing and visual impairment)
Know about different types of communication breakdown
Be aware of and reflect on nursing home communication barriers (lack of time, lack of opportunity, task-focused and ignoring communication, elder speak)
Correct misconceptions about communication with people with dementia. Learn about basic concepts of communication with people with dementia such as basal stimulation, the validation approach, and person-centred care
Maximize your own skills to maximize communication potential

Eggenberger et al. surmise the communication skills training sessions they reviewed do result in positive outcomes; "Professional and family caregivers' communication skills, competencies, and knowledge significantly increases compared to those in non-intervention conditions" (Eggenberger et al, 2013, p. 13). In making this statement they provide some warning, however, that these approaches must not be delivered as single doses but require some ongoing input to help staff to apply the new skills they have learned. Yet single-dose training approaches are frequently both the maximum amount that commissioners are willing to pay for and that staff are able to attend. Indeed, it is not always possible for staff who work weekend or night shifts to attend training led by an SLT somewhere between 9.00 in the morning and 5.00 in the afternoon, Monday to Fridays.

Communication skills training is typically delivered in person and requires significant time away from clinical work for both trainers (SLTs) and trainees (typically nurses, medical and other healthcare staff). A recent study by Heard, O'Halloran and McKinley (2017) compared the effectiveness of two methods of delivering training, one of which incorporated an online e-learning session. Online learning is becoming increasingly popular in health care but not everybody feels this medium delivers the same effectiveness of learning and skill development. The first intervention in the study by Heard et al. (2017) used the Supported Conversation for Adults with Aphasia, SCA[TM] programme (Kagan et al., 2001) and was delivered over two 90-minute face-to-face sessions using the SCA[TM] materials. During these sessions, the trainer provided information on aphasia and strategies that can support communication, as well as opportunities for role play and practice. The second programme was delivered by one 30-minute e-learning session and one 60-minute face-to-face session. Sixty-four healthcare staff were recruited and randomly assigned to each programme. Both groups demonstrated similar improvements in knowledge and confidence post-education session. Importantly the e-learning package was found to cost less in terms of resources. The researchers emphasize the need to consider innovative online training approaches that cost less to ensure staff are able to access communication skills training, so they in turn can support people with communication needs at any time of day or night. Delivering training via online and e-learning mediums is inevitable in our current IT-savvy climate, and research demonstrating its effectiveness is valuable to justify this.

Time and resources are not the only barrier to this type of training. SLTs who read this will not be surprised that there is far more evidence around training nurses and care staff than medical staff. That is not to say medical staff do not need this type of training. Unfortunately, there are frequently some additional institutional- and resource-led barriers that prevent these professionals accessing communication skills training. This emphasizes the need to explore briefer, more accessible, practical training techniques and their effectiveness. Saldert, Forsgren and Hartelius (2016) describe how a speech and language therapy department at the University of Gothenburg in Sweden trialled a new approach to teaching medical students. Fifty-nine undergraduate medical students received a 45-minute lecture on speech and language disorders. Twenty-six of these medical students also went on to participate in a workshop which included demonstrations of communication aids and interacting with students SLTs (who had been trained to act as people with stroke-related aphasia or Parkinson's disease). In these role-play situations, medical students practised using the communication strategies they were learning about. All 59 medical students were asked to complete a rating scale that included rating their own confidence in supporting communication, their knowledge of suitable strategies and their attitude to people with communication difficulties. The results demonstrated more improvements in confidence, knowledge and a change in attitude in the medical students who had received the additional workshop. This is not surprising when one considers the previous discussion that has emphasized the need for practical follow-up to maximize the mastery of practical skills in conversation.

In a subsequent study the same researchers examined the outcomes of this type of training in more detail (Forsgren, Hartelius, & Saldert, 2017). Similar to the previous study they trained a large cohort of medical students in a lecture and selected 36 to attend a further two-and-a-half-hour workshop where they received further training in communication strategies and participated in role play and discussions. Both groups were asked to complete a questionnaire and, in addition, students who attended the workshop were video-recorded having simulated conversations with people with communication difficulties prior to and following the workshop activities. Recordings were analyzed, and desired communication strategies coded and counted for comparison. As previously, the results of the study demonstrated more improvements in confidence, knowledge and ability to identify relevant strategies among the students who had attended the workshop. Analysis of video data also demonstrated specific improvements in the use of supportive strategies; particularly encouraging people with communication difficulties to use gestures, pointing, a calendar and use of writing. The authors highlight the value of experiential learning to develop skills in the use of communication strategies.

These studies demonstrate that to genuinely benefit from communication skills training attendees required more than a didactic lecture-style intervention. Even brief opportunities to practise and problem-solve the use of communication strategies are helpful. Creative opportunities such as role play and using SLT students in these sessions produced tangible changes in skill.

Communication training for capacity: The evidence

The studies described so far provide examples of approaches to communication training that may be useful when planning your own sessions, yet they do not directly address decision making and mental capacity. There are few examples in the research literature of communication training for professionals that aims specifically to support people in issues related to decision making. Simmons-Mackie et al. (2007) and Carling-Rowland et al. (2014) are two rare but useful examples. It is important to note that both these studies were based in Canada where legislation differs to the UK, but still the research they report is useful and relevant to the field of speech and language therapy.

The first study by Simmons-Mackie et al. (2007) was based on the notion that the ultimate goal is improved communication access "in the larger realm of society or systems" (p.41) and thus a top-down approach is required to target these systems. The researchers describe a qualitative study examining the effectiveness of a multidisciplinary communication skills training programme that they developed for three groups of health professionals working with people with aphasia. The training aimed to improve communication access to information and decision making for people with aphasia. To achieve maximum buy-in they invited the managers at each organization (an acute hospital, a rehabilitation centre and a long-term care facility) to select a team to participate in the project, with a requirement that the managers also participate in the process themselves. Consequently, the participants attended a two-day training session and received post-training follow-up and support for four months to enable them to make genuine changes in their work places.

The two-day training was based on Supported Conversation for Aphasia TM (SCA) training methods (Kagan, 1998) and included: (1) information about aphasia; (2) hands-on experience in using Supported Conversation, focusing on access to information and decision making for people with aphasia; (3) brainstorming about access issues within their facilities; (4) selection of facility-specific goals designed to enhance communicative access. During the follow-up phase, teams were supported to develop and produce individualized support resources by a project SLT who visited them on site to discuss and problem-solve the implementation of these ideas. The SLT attended team meetings, provided material resources and spoke to managers or team members on the telephone when any help was needed.

Before and after taking part in the project trainees participated in interviews and focus groups. These were analyzed using thematic analysis techniques. Results highlighted that all trainees and trainee groups felt there had been tangible improvements in their knowledge, skills and daily practice, although the staff group from the acute setting identified significantly more barriers. Examples of these included a lack of support from senior medical colleagues (who had not attended the training), a need for timely interactions, and the medical model that dominates in the acute healthcare setting. In the rehabilitation and long-term care facility there were significant improvements in staff's understanding of service users' needs and their ability to reduce these barriers. They reported that before training they preferred to 'terminate' interactions if a person with aphasia was having difficulties, or make decisions for them without asking. After training, participants reported creative methods of modifying their own communication. One group set a goal to develop an accessible consent form and implemented it as standard practice in their facility.

Simmons-Mackie et al. (2007)'s example of communication training endeavours to bridge many of the gaps identified by Eggenberger et al.'s systematic review – namely follow-up is key to carryover and implementation, with involvement of senior staff members to endorse and encourage participation. Yet barriers in culture within organizations can be difficult to change; the paternalistic medical model being one of the most challenging. This, and other issues such as staff sickness and team morale are often more complex and beyond the scope of a one-off training event, but require a lengthy and multi-pronged approach.

Another significant, and extremely useful, piece of work around communication skills training for capacity assessors was carried out in Canada by Carling-Rowland et al. (2014). The Ontario Ministry of Health and Long-Term Care (1997) developed a tool entitled *The Capacity to Make Admissions Decisions* (CMAD), an assessment of decision-making capacity for admission to long-term care. In this study, Carling-Rowland et al. describe how they developed and validated an accessible version of the CMAD called the Communication Aid to Capacity Evaluation (CACE). The researchers consequently conducted a randomized controlled trial with 32 social workers who were each paired with a person with aphasia. All were asked to assess the person's decision-making capacity using the original local tool; the CMAD. Half of the social workers were then trained to use the CACE tool using a training DVD. After a two-week interval, all the social work participants were then asked to re-assess the people with aphasia. At this point the group of social workers who had participated in the training used the CACE tool. Results showed that the social workers who had been trained had significantly better communication skills and were better able to accurately assess the capacity of the individuals with aphasia. They were able to 'reveal their competence' in decision making using the skills they had learned.

The 37-minute training DVD developed by Carling-Rowland et al. (2014) is freely available on the internet at the following web address (and on YouTube): https://www.aphasia.ca/home-page/health-care-professionals/resources-and-tools/cace/. The training DVD presents a person with moderate-to-severe Broca's aphasia speaking with an SLT. First the SLT assesses him with the local CMAD tool, without any communication support. The DVD then presents the SLT assessing the person again, using the CACE and supportive communication strategies. The video explains and highlights these strategies as they are used. The CACE tool itself is also available to download. The CACE has been designed to be accessible for people with aphasia and has images and diagrams to support explanations and content. It is accompanied by communication cards and supplementary information to support the assessment.

As mentioned, the training DVD is freely available as is the CACE tool, together with helpful additional resources such as the communication cards. It may be useful to use some aspects of these freely-available tools in the UK, being mindful of the fact that they have been designed for a Canadian audience where the capacity legislation is different to here. Perhaps the most useful aspects are the video vignettes. However, rather than sending these out in advance of a training session, it would be advisable to use these as part of your own training so the information relating to Canadian legislation and assessment processes is not misconstrued.

Table 5.2 makes some suggestions around the activities and content of training sessions. In particular there are references and links to video clips, made in England, demonstrating the positive impact of supporting communication made by the charity organization Dyscover (not during a capacity assessment as such but nevertheless demonstrating the impact of accessible communication in revealing an individual's competence). Many third-sector organizations have made videos explaining what conditions such as aphasia and dementia

Table 5.2 Suggestions of activities and content for group communication training in relation to decision-making and the Mental Capacity Act (MCA, 2005).

Approach	Activity
Pre-training information Consider recommending pre-training reading or activities for attendees	Recommending attendees read an article on the communication needs of their particular speciality, or a set of guidelines (perhaps a local policy) on communication support that should be implemented, could be useful. Even just asking them to identify the relevant section of the MCA re communication could be helpful. Alternatively, you may choose to send them a chapter in a book (such as this book), or photocopy Table 5.1 which summarizes Eggenberger et al.'s (2012) findings from the systematic review. This could form a useful prompt card or tick sheet for attendees. Sending something more interactive may be more engaging; you could send out a link to a lecture or online training package. It is not unusual in large organizations to have online training modules. These are often used as a method of establishing a baseline knowledge prior to more interactive training. Does your organization have one already that you can use? Platforms such as YouTube provide great opportunities for uploading your own video (you could make and send out a video of yourself delivering a brief lecture summarizing the common communication disorders and strategies that can support this); alternatively you can search for existing online materials. There are charity organizations, such as Dyscover, that provide a useful set of videos. The first is most useful in illustrating the impact that using communication strategies can have in supporting people in conversation: https://www.youtube.com/watch?v=KWVoqM9jmEM https://www.youtube.com/watch?v=zS5aRSfE1XI https://www.youtube.com/watch?v=U5u1Q8KZP40 This Australian charity has produced a video on tips for communicating with people with aphasia: https://www.youtube.com/watch?v=aPTTjRTmgq0 This is a really useful illustrated explanation of how aphasia works: https://www.youtube.com/watch?v=-GsVhbmecJA Speakability (a charity) has also produced some useful video clips explaining what aphasia is: https://www.youtube.com/watch?v=XYXSxNu01gc Asking people to bring a case study to discuss or asking them to bring any tools they know of or use to support communication can prove useful.

(Continued over)

| **Content of training session** Consider using both educational and practical skill-based activities that address the following stages: 1. Understand the communi-cation difficulty 2. Understand how this relates to mental capacity 3. Understand what can reduce these barriers 4. Be able to confidently use the strategies 5. Actually use them. | Start by introducing yourself and your interest in this area. Making it personal if it is a small group can help to build rapport rapidly. Introduce learning outcomes (see Chapter 8 on evaluation) and timing for the session to support expectations. It may be useful to start communication training by breaking communication down into the components we require to understand a single spoken word: Need to be able to hear it / Differentiate it from other sounds (cars/animals) / Know it is a language we understand / Recognise the word / Have the word in our dictionary of meanings Or the components to say a single word: Know what we want to say / Know the word that goes with it / Know the sounds that that word has / Send the motor plan for that word to our muscles / Make the muscles move properly Or the components to participate in a conversation: Understand more than one word / Understand grammar / Remember all that is being said / Know when to take a turn / Attend to the conversation and stay on topic / Know what is appropriate and not appropriate / Plan an idea and initiate that idea. You could do this using a brainstorm, or by presenting a visual diagram. Using a visual diagram can help people break this process up. 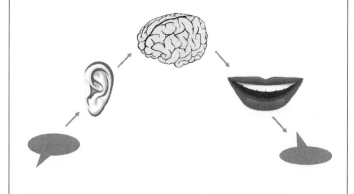 |

It may be useful to include definitions of different communication difficulties.

The definitions

Dysarthria – weakness, loss of range, loss of co-ordination of muscle movements (Speech)

Dyspraxia – Difficulties in programming muscle movements (Speech)

Dysphasia – language impairment (phonological, semantics, syntax, grammar)

Dysphonia – loss of voice

Dysphagia – swallowing difficulties

CCD- cognitive communication difficulties

Linking these to their causes, e.g., stroke, dementia, etc., may be useful and thus linking this to the MCA can help illustrate the relevance of communication difficulties to working with people who may lack capacity.

Depending on the level of detail you are planning to provide you may wish to present examples of exactly what these communication difficulties mean: video recordings of people with aphasia, or apraxia or example picture descriptions from testing, e.g., cookie theft picture descriptions.

This can be linked with case studies or real service user examples where you present a person who has a brain impairment, their consequent communication difficulties and how it presents.

Describing how communication difficulties affect decision making can be helpful. This could be done as a brainstorming activity or by presenting the relevant evidence in this area:

Understanding, retention, weighing up and communicating decisions

- People with dementia (even mild) often failed an assessment on **understanding** (Moye et al, 2007).

- People with Alzheimer's dementia who had difficulties with conceptualisation, verbal fluency and naming demonstrated difficulties in **understanding, appreciating and reasoning** related to a medical decision (Moye et al, 2007).

- People with Parkinson's dementia who had executive difficulties and memory impairments demonstrated most difficulty in **understanding and reasoning** related to a decision (Moye et al, 2007).

- People with mild brain injury are most impaired in the domain of **understanding**, whilst people with moderate and severe brain injuries are impaired across all domains (Triebel et al, 2012). Improvement over 6 months with weighing up being most long lasting area of difficulty (Marson et al, 2005).

(Continued over)

To increase people's understanding and empathy it can be useful to provide an experience of how communication affects decision making. Practical tasks can be very helpful here:

Ask people to get into pairs and for one person to verbally (no gestures) explain how they are going to put a plaster on a cut without using the word 'cut' or 'plaster'. Afterwards ask the listener what they understood was about to happen. Did this person understand?

Ask one person in the pair to explain the same thing without using any words (nonverbally). Afterwards ask the listener what they understood. Did this person understand?

Ask people to reflect on their experiences of other languages, for example how they chose what to buy from a delicatessen in another country when they didn't understand and were unable to use the language.

Ask people to reflect on when they have themselves been unwell and lost their voice/had a cold that affected their hearing and how this has felt.

Ask people how they managed when they were in a noisy pub or at party and couldn't hear anyone; how did they overcome the barriers to communication.

(These last three suggestions lead nicely into the next stage)

Then consider how you can maximize communication. This is where the video clips from Dyscover or the Canadian CACE resources may be useful to demonstrate the impact of supported communication.

It may also be useful to ask attendees to share their existing knowledge of communication strategies. Sharing strategies in this way can ensure contributors feel empowered by their existing knowledge, and can highlight that strategy use is achievable for others.

You can also present information on methods of supporting communication by providing checklists or prompt cards with information on, for example:

What helps communication:

Verbal strategies
Repetition
Use one step instructions or statements
One question or statement at a time
Give time to process (pause)
Use pitch and intonation to emphasize key words

Nonverbal strategies
Communication aids will help
Writing drawing
Gesture
Pointing or demonstrating
Showing what you mean

	At this point it is useful to start consolidating this through practice. You can:
	Perform a vignette for the group; using poor communication, ask them how it could be done better and then re-do the scenario with the ideas from the group.
	Ask people to get into pairs, ask one person to act as a person with communication difficulties, ask the other to assess their decision-making capacity to have an operation.
	Ask student SLTs to help, to act as a person with communication difficulties
	Ask past service users to attend to give attendees the experience of working with real communication difficulties in imaginary scenarios
	Ask trainees to identify the barriers to implementing these strategies in assessments of decision making. These may be easy to identify in a brainstorming session or by using case studies to illustrate different situations (people may be invited to bring difficult examples with them, or you could provide some examples).
	Ask trainees to identify potential solutions to these barriers – they may know some solutions but find it difficult to address or implement them.
	It can be valuable to finish a with a reflection:
	A thank you, where each person says thank-you for something specific to do with the session, or chooses a picture from a selection that they feel best represents their experience in the group and then explains or shares it with the group
	Asking participants to identify one thing that they have learned or one thing they will do to change their practice, and write it down or announce it to the group
Post-training follow-up Consider planning a post-training activity that embeds the use of	Setting homework or an assignment may feel rather excessive, but this could be something as simple as asking all attendees to report back to you about a strategy they use the next time they support someone in their communication.
	Mentoring or role modelling can be really useful and very practical. If you have the time and resources it may be worth visiting trainees individually and supporting them in their practice. Modelling communication strategies in a joint session, and giving feedback on an individual's performance, may aid in consolidating and increasing confidence.
	Follow-up meetings and case discussions, when specific issues arise, can be practical too.
	Supporting trainees to address specific issues where they work may be useful. Invite them to identify something they would like to improve, make suggestions on how they can implement change, provide them with materials or resources and support them through this. Act as project advisor – empowering them to actually implement change.
	Some organizations choose to encourage annual refreshers and updates. This may or may not be appropriate for the staff group you work with.

are, and have posted them online so they are freely available. You may find it useful to search for the most relevant examples for the people and population you work with.

Development of training: Piloting

Being mindful of the lack of evidence doesn't mean it is not possible to plan and deliver a relevant and effective training session. It is appropriate in these situations to use evidence from practice-based knowledge and transfer our knowledge of what works in other areas, looking to some of the literature summarized above. Looking back to the development and evaluation process in Figure 5.2, the next step would be to pilot the training you have developed. Ideally, piloting would happen before you continue to deliver the training more widely. This might mean that the first training session you deliver would act as the pilot. At this point, you may choose to tweak and amend things before you continue to deliver and evaluate further training sessions. When piloting the training the following questions may be helpful:

- Was the content useful (both pre-training information and training itself)?

- Did trainees have any suggestions or want to change things?

- Did the session work as planned: Did you do everything in the time frame? Did the slides work? Did the video work? Did the practice tasks work? Did people attend the session?

Realistically, piloting a programme such as this in a clinical setting may not be achievable, but running the programme past a colleague or doing a dry run (of elements of the programme or the entire programme) without the trainees present might be helpful. It is likely that piloting, evaluation and implementation will overlap significantly. Unless you are developing a rigorous intervention programme that you are planning to use for research purposes, ongoing modification and tweaking to meet the needs of each individual cohort is appropriate. Thus, evaluating the effectiveness of the training may be more about what the trainees, commissioners and you need, rather than the effectiveness (see Chapter 8 on evaluation). And implementation of change in communication may be constrained by trainees, commissioners and your own time and resources. Thus, any training you do deliver may be limited by any number of these factors. Recognizing these limitations is useful, and addressing them where you are able and this is achievable will contribute to continually improving your training and consequently the practice of the trainees. This process cycle is illustrated in Figures 5.1 and 5.2.

Communication skills training for individuals and their conversation partner

> "The fact that conversation is a collaborative event suggests that both parties require skills and often the skills are dyad dependent" (Simmons-Mackie et al., 2014, p. 522)

Communication skills training in large organizations is often designed to address the healthcare professional's skills, and sometimes the family's skills, rather than the individual with the communication difficulty. Although this top-down approach is no doubt important and effective in reducing the systematic and societal barriers to communication for people with communication difficulties, as evidenced by the above discussion, there are some situations that require a more person-centred and individualized approach. Indeed, there are situations where working with the person alone, or with them and their caregiver together, may be preferable. Communication skills training may be delivered in one-off sessions to family or professionals; equally, this type of training may be delivered over a number of sessions of therapy intervention.

In this context, Simmons-Mackie et al. (2014) have developed a very useful framework that can assist in conceptualizing the exact approach you are planning to take in communication skills training. They conducted a qualitative review of the research literature on conversation therapy in aphasia. By definition, this incorporated interventions that may also be called communication skills training approaches, approaches to communication support and interaction-focused therapies. In their review, Simmons-Mackie et al. define conversation therapy as "direct, planned therapy that is designed to enhance conversational skill and confidence using activities that directly address conversation *and* focus on changing behaviours within the context of genuine conversation" (Simmons-Mackie et al., 2014, p. 512).

After searching databases for articles that met their inclusion criteria and definition of conversation therapy, Simmons-Mackie et al. identified 30 articles for inclusion. They used thematic analysis techniques to systematically code the content of the studies and consequently identified key themes. These themes resulted in a descriptive taxonomy that can help to characterize and contrast key elements of conversation therapy. Although this taxonomy arose from the aphasia literature, many aspects are equally relevant to people with a variety of communication difficulties including cognitive communication difficulties, dementia and motor speech disorders. And although this review did not contrast and compare the effectiveness of these interventions it is certainly a useful framework for considering and critiquing the key components of such an intervention. Further, this taxonomy (which can be found in the published article) is a useful tool for clinicians planning communication skills training sessions..

Simmons-Mackie et al. (2014) explain the key components of conversation therapy in this taxonomy and thus the key aspects to consider when planning and developing such an intervention (the following provides a summary of each domain):

Therapy participants: Who is actually participating in the therapy sessions? The research literature in this area includes interventions targeting the person with the communication difficulties, or their communication partners or both (the 'dyad' or 'couple'). There is evidence that each of these approaches may be effective in improving the skills of the participants and reducing barriers to participation – and thus decision making. Specifically, there are a selection of effective dyadic interventions described in the research literature that can be useful to consult, such as: Conversational Coaching (Hopper, Holland, & Rewega, 2002); Interaction-Focused Therapy (Wilkinson, Lock, Bryan, & Sage, 2011); and Communication Partner Training (CPT) (e.g., Blom Johansson et al.. 2013, Saldert, backman, & Hartelius, 2013); Supporting Partners of People with Aphasia in Relationships and Conversation (SPPARC), and Better Conversations with Aphasia (BCA, Beeke et al., 2013), also Better Conversations with Primary Progressive Aphasia (BCPPA, Volkmer et al., forthcoming 2019).

Principal roots: Conversation therapy interventions draw on a variety of philosophical, theoretical or practical origins. Life participation is an approach that draws on social or participation models of intervention, and focuses directly on enhancing engagement in life situations. Functional, behavioural orientations draw on practice-based knowledge and the experience of SLTs, and are based on practical approaches. Conversation analysis (CA) is a rigorous approach to analyzing natural conversation that focuses on structural features such as turn taking and repairing communicative breakdowns. Counselling-oriented approaches explicitly incorporate elements drawn from the counselling literature.

Mode of service delivery: Conversation therapy may be delivered in individual therapy where the SLT works with one person or one dyad, or in group therapy with a number of individuals (people with aphasia or conversation partners or dyads).

Focus of intervention: Conversation therapy may be delivered using a generic agenda or tailored to meet the individual needs of those being trained. The intervention itself may focus on addressing and eliminating problems in conversation or teaching solutions. Generally, all approaches focus on compensatory strategies to improve interactions.

Methods: The training approaches themselves can be described on a spectrum ranging from ones that are explicit – overtly discussing and naming behaviours, strategies and goals that are being worked on – versus implicit training at the other end of the spectrum where modelling and mediating is pursued without actually instructing people in specific skills. Explicit approaches often involve education, discussion, role-play and video examples to build awareness of particular behaviours as a prerequisite to behavioural change.

Further consideration may be given to whether the instructions or education component happen outside of the actual conversation, or occur during a real-time conversational context; embedded in the interaction.

Simmons-Mackie et al. (2014) describe a range of methods used to enhance conversational skill or participation in the training sessions (see Table 5.3).

Outcome measures: Finally, Simmons-Mackie et al. (2014) describe the outcome measures used in these interventions as ranging widely from conversation analysis as an outcome, specific measurement of discrete behaviours, use of rating scales, interviews and questionnaires or social validity judgements. Simmons-Mackie et al.'s qualitative review of the key elements of the research literature on conversation therapies does not focus on effectiveness, nor does it focus explicitly on access to decision making.

Table 5.3 Examples of methods employed to change conversational skill or participation from Simmons-Mackie et al. (2014, p.520).

Using supports for message transmission
- Communicative drawing (Lyon, 1995)
- Gestures
- Writing
- Vocalization, facial expression, body language
- Graphic choices or written key words (Garrett & Beukelman, 1995; Kagan & Gailey, 1993)
- Pictographs, visual scenes or photographs
- Technology
- Use of other material resources (communication books, rating scales, maps, 'props' such as magazines)

Facilitating 'routinised' elements of conversation
- Scripting (Elman & Bernstein-Ellis, 1999, Youmans et al., 2005)

Practising specific skills
- Role play (Kagan,1998)
- Engaging in 'creative' communication (e.g., mime, Elman & Bernstein-Ellis, 1999; theatre, Cherney et al., 2011)
- Video recognition and substitution training (identifying problem behaviours and monitoring implementation of a new skill) (Simmons-Mackie et al., 1987, 2005)

Promoting conversational participation
- Asking the person with aphasia to lead a topic or share the facilitator role in a group (Elman & Bernstein-Ellis, 1999).
- Clinician using gaze and silence to encourage the participation of the person with aphasia (Simmons-Mackie et al., 2007a; Simmons-Mackie & Damico, 2009)

Educational 'external' methods
- Defining and demonstrating behaviours or elements of conversation in general, or problem behaviours specific to individuals or dyads (Kagan 1998; Lock et al., 2001a, 2001b)
- Handouts
- Lectures
- Discussions
- Video examples
- Role play

Embedded methods used while engaging in conversation
- Mediating meanings
- Scaffolding
- Modelling
- Reinforcing target behaviours within the context of conversation
- Coaching (e.g., pointing out a potential strategy)

Communication training for individuals and communication partners focused on decision making and mental capacity: The evidence

Having considered the key elements of your training approach, described above, it is also useful to consider any specific examples of communication training to support decision-making capacity from the research literature. Unfortunately, there is a paucity of research literature in the area of communication training and decision making but what is there focuses on both individualized training (for the professional or carer) and training for both the service user and the communication partner. There are some studies that focus on communication training for joint decision making in a medical setting or at the end-of-life in cancer care. The examples discussed in this chapter do not focus on working with people with communication difficulties per se, but include useful elements that we can learn from. There are also some SLT-focused communication training programmes that focus on or include decision making. Looking to both of these sources may provide useful guidance.

Kruser et al. (2017) attempted to improve joint decision making with older adults in complex surgical situations. They developed a novel communication tool called 'Best Case/Worst Case' (BC/WC), a pen-and-paper aid that illustrates two or more treatment choices. This was accompanied by a two-hour training session so surgeons could use the aid in their consultation to tell a story about how the service user might experience the surgery outcomes. This included discussion of the best- and worst-case scenarios, estimation of the most likely outcome, and providing a treatment recommendation.

Kruser et al. (2017) describe using the BC/WC tool in a pilot study where 25 surgeons attended a group training session before they participated in individual practice and feedback sessions with a coach observing them. This included a 15-minute lecture highlighting the essential tool elements, followed by a demonstration with a service user. After this, each surgeon practised using the tool with two simulated cases observed by a coach who provided online one-to-one feedback during and after the first simulation. Results of the study reported that surgeons felt the tool was an improvement on usual care and that they continued to use the tool, whilst service users reported that clearer information was presented when their surgeons used the tool in the discussion. This creative approach combined the time-saving benefits of group training with the benefits of individualized one-to-one practice and feedback.

Another creative approach combined training both the professionals, on the one hand, and the person and their family, on the other, to participate in shared decision making at the end of life, and comes from the cancer literature. Epstein et al. (2017) recognize that making high-quality conversations happen is difficult at the best of times, highlighting barriers held by both parties. In particular, the service users are often reluctant to ask questions, express emotions directly, or state opinions and preferences (Epstein et al., 2017). These researchers therefore recognized the positive effects of training both parties and endeavoured to maximize the impact by combining them in a randomized trial. Both interventions emphasized how to engage service users to participate in the consultation, respond to their emotions, inform them about prognosis and treatment choices, and provide information in a balanced manner. The trainers chose to go directly to the professionals; delivering two 45-minute sessions of 'in-office' training to oncologists randomized to the treatment arm. This included a brief 15-minute education video and personalized feedback from up to two audio recorded consultations. Service users and their partners participated in a single one-hour coaching session incorporating a question prompt list to help identify their concerns with their oncologist plus up to three follow-up phone calls. The authors report meaningful increases in balanced discussions, responses to emotions and explanations of prognosis and treatment choices as well as improvements in oncologists' empathy and service user-reported trust when compared to the control group. This novel and creative treatment approach again seeks to overcome the barriers faced by many professionals working in hectic, medically-driven roles by visiting them in their office, at their convenience and providing tailored brief interventions.

These interventions have primarily targeted health professionals, yet many family caregivers are responsible for daily decision making when involved in care giving. These are frequently the most difficult decisions for caregivers, even if they have been donated power of attorney and are involved in making significant decisions about health, welfare and financial affairs. Samsi and Manthorpe (2013) conducted qualitative research with the family carers of people with dementia about everyday decision making; specifically, how decisions were negotiated and how this changed. They held face-to-face interviews with participants approximately four times over the course of a year. Findings from the study reported that carers expressed concerns about the level of responsibility in making decisions for their loved ones, and found it a strain. Some did develop their own strategies (for example asking people at 'the right time') but only a few carers reported receiving support in this; most carers reported they would benefit from support in decision making but this was not really available.

Some of the most difficult decisions that carers have to make are related to daily living activities such as cooking, washing, shopping, etc. These decisions are often complicated by feelings of guilt, where carers endeavour to maintain maximum levels of independence yet keep loved ones safe. Daily care can be difficult to discuss and disagreements can be distressing and add to the perceived burden of care. As dementia progressively affects both cognition and communication it can become increasingly difficult to support interaction between people with dementia and their carers. Murphy and Oliver (2013) describe using a low-technology communication framework, Talking Mats©, to help couples in this situation.

Talking Mats© was designed to support people with communication difficulties to express their views. Using a simple system of picture symbols and a visual scale placed on a textured mat, people indicate their feelings about various options within a topic. Murphy and Oliver (2013) examined whether Talking Mats© could support family carers and people with dementia to discuss issues around daily living. Eighteen couples (people with dementia and their family carers) from Scotland and the North of England were recruited to the study. The researcher visited each of the couples at home and facilitated two discussions both focusing on personal care, getting around, housework and daily activities. Couples were asked to discuss the topics either using their usual method of communication or using the Talking Mats© framework. Half of the couples used Talking Mats© at their first visit, and usual communication at the next; half of the couples completed the discussions in reverse (usual communication first and Talking Mats© second). At the end of the Talking Mats© discussion, a photograph was taken of the mat as a record for the couple and later analysis. After the couples had completed the study each participant was asked to complete a short questionnaire to assess how involved they felt in each discussion. Results of the study demonstrated that all of the participants felt more involved when using Talking Mats© than when using their usual method of communication. Participants reported a reduction in confrontation and arguments using images that supported memory and language within the discussion. People with dementia reported that Talking Mats© helped to clarify their thoughts and enabled them to express their views. Family carers reported feeling more satisfied with the outcome when using Talking Mats©, stating that it allowed a better understanding of the views of the person with dementia. The researchers summarized that the Talking Mats© framework not only allowed the people with dementia to convey their thoughts to their family carers and contributed to the process of negotiation in day-to-day decision making, but also offered a method for recording views to inform later decision making.

Although not a training approach itself per se, people benefit from training and support in using Talking Mats©. More importantly Murphy and Oliver's (2013) work demonstrates the potential positive impact that communication aids can have in facilitating discussion around decision making for people and their family caregivers. Murphy and her colleagues have conducted a number of studies demonstrating the effectiveness of using Talking Mats© with different client groups in daily conversations.

Communication aids are a useful approach to supporting people in discussions around difficult decision making, and training people to use these tools is invaluable. Previously, Volkmer (2016) has advocated the benefit of including advance health and care decisions in communication books and aids. Yet unless couples are both trained and supported to use these tools people may not be able to take advantage of them in order to maintain their voice in their healthcare decisions.

Better Conversations with Aphasia (BCA, UCLeXtend website) was originally developed as a free online conversation training tool for SLTs to use with people with non-progressive language difficulties and their conversation partners. It has been demonstrated to increase the use of facilitators and reduce the number of barriers in a conversation with people with non-progressive aphasia (Beeke et al., 2014, 2015; Best et al., 2016) through a series of sessions whereby the couple reflect on video recordings of their own conversations and are supported to identify specific barriers and facilitators impacting on the effectiveness of their conversations. Using BCA the SLT supports the couple to set goals, and to practise and implement these changes in their conversations.

More recently, work has commenced on a Better Conversations with Primary Progressive Aphasia (BCPPA, Volkmer et al., forthcoming) programme. In the process of refining the original tool to meet the needs of people with PPA, the researchers explored what SLTs and people living with PPA wanted the tool to address. As a result of this work (a consensus group exercise and a series of focus groups with people with PPA and their families), it was identified that people wanted the intervention to incorporate an element of future planning around decision making (Volkmer, Spector, & Beeke, 2018). The final session of the programme emphasizes the need for the SLT to support people to continue reflecting and modifying communication strategies as language deteriorates in the condition. It also addresses future decision making and provides prompts to sourcing information on power of attorney and advance

Table 5.4 Suggestions of activities and content for individual or dyad focused communication training in relation to decision-making and the MCA.

Approach	Activity
Pre-therapy: Collecting information on the areas of communication breakdown	Ask the participants to self-rate their conversation prior to therapy. You could also ask them to rate one another's communication, or ask a colleague or service user to rate their communication skills. This rating scale can be very simple to develop yourself, or you might choose to use published rating scales relevant to the specific people you are working with. You may equally choose to use the articles described above as a source; Murphy and Oliver, 2013, for example, include the questions they asked their participants in their journal article.
	Using a case study (from Chapter 2 in this book) might be a useful tool when asking professionals to reflect on what they would do next. You could do this before and after training. This may be done face-to-face, or written down. Equally, this approach may be appropriate for certain family caregivers. Asking people for examples of where communication has broken down in their own lives and exactly what happened could serve a similar purpose.
	Observing an individual's communication skills in action can be a useful method of identifying areas of breakdown. This may be more acceptable in some ways, as health professionals are often used to being observed, although this doesn't allow the individuals themselves to see and reflect on their own communication.
	Audio or video recording a conversation or interaction is another more permanent record and can support people to reflect on their own communication. This data may be more challenging to collect, but both mediums are becoming increasing more accessible and acceptable using handheld devices, mobile telephones, etc.
	Having identified the area of communication breakdown you will be better prepared to tailor the intervention to meet an individual's needs.
Training sessions	A degree of education and information is useful, often as a framework to proceed with the intervention. This may include a formal explanation of the communication aid or tool you are introducing, or a formal education on the structure of conversation, e.g., the concepts of turn taking, topic maintenance, breakdown and repair, and how this structure works in practice. Using handouts and more didactic methods may be helpful here. Both of the Better Conversations programmes (BCA and BCPPA) provide freely-available handouts to download from the internet.
	It is valuable to include examples at this point, before embarking on a practice session. This could include a demonstration of the tool or aid you are introducing, in the context of how this may support decision making. It may be helpful to have readily available video recordings of the tools in action. The video examples from Dyscover, CACE and so forth summarized in Table 5.2 may prove useful. There are a number of video recordings available on YouTube demonstrating Talking Mats© in action. The Better Conversations programmes also include video examples of communication breakdown and facilitators. Ideally, video recordings of the people you are working with would be useful to use at this point.

(Continued over)

	Practice is always important. This can be usefully guided by setting a specific goal or aim for the period of practice. For example:
	To present the decision to be made using total communication strategies
	To use Talking Mats© when discussing decisions related to certain a situation
	To observe X's nonverbal communication during a conversation about a decision and check what it means with X
	To ask X questions about their opinion on the decision when presenting information related to the issue in hand
	To give X time to ask questions during a conversation related to a decision
	Practice tasks would ideally involve simulated or genuine discussions related to decision making. This may be achieved by providing people with topics or scenarios to discuss, or by asking them to generate their own. Discussing small decisions such as what a couple may wish to purchase as a gift for someone, or what activity they may like to do tomorrow, may be a useful start.
	Equally, supporting a discussion on difficult subjects should not be avoided in the training itself, so discussing funeral arrangements, future healthcare decisions, financial issues and so forth may be productively broached in the training sessions.
	Problem solving should not be avoided. It is not easy to implement a new strategy or tool immediately, and to use it perfectly. Individuals should be given the opportunity for repeated practice, homework assignments (having discussions outside of training) and consequently fine tuning these with support.
Follow-up	As the training finishes it would be worth incorporating a specific commitment to continue using the strategies learned in future conversations related to decision making. This may include reporting back to the SLT, telephone follow-up, or refresher training/re-referral at particular points when further input may be required.

decision making. At the time of writing, BCPPA is currently being piloted across a number of National Health Service (NHS) sites (Volkmer, Warren, Spector, et al., in press) and is due to be launched in the next two years as a free online programme for SLTs, hosted by the UCLeXtend website. This work really emphasizes that people living with communication difficulties, their families and SLTs have identified a need for tools and materials to support decision making and mental capacity.

Table 5.4 provides suggestions and activities for individual- or dyad-focused communication training in relation to decision making and the MCA based on the research literature reviewed in this chapter as well as additional ideas.

Conclusion

There are a small number of accessible tools and training programmes that can support SLTs in delivering evidence-based and effective communication training to health and social care professionals, as well as family and people living with communication difficulties themselves. There is a paucity of research examining the effectiveness of communication training methods that specifically address decision making and mental capacity. Having reviewed the research literature in these areas there are certainly overlaps, and clinically it is justifiable to borrow and tweak tools to meet the needs of the individuals you are working with.

In reality, the training we are doing around communication skills does not and will not reach all professionals and people we wish it to reach. McCormick, Bose and Marinis (2017) found that SLTs report training mostly (in this order) occupational therapists, physiotherapists, nursing staff, healthcare assistants, doctors, relatives and carers to support people with aphasia in decision making. In terms of referrals seeking support in these cases it seems quite the reverse, with the majority of referrals coming from (in this order) consultants, social workers, occupational therapists, and physiotherapists. This highlights the presence of potential barriers (both institutional, resource-based and attitudinal) to training professionals in this area – it seems the consultants and social workers may benefit most, yet are not receiving the training.

In preparing any type of training it is likely you will encounter some such barriers and it is worth considering well in advance what these might be and any possible solutions in the process. Consulting with service users can often shed light on the issues at hand, and can ensure what you develop is relevant (see Chapter 7). In addition, focusing on the evaluation – the trainees' needs – in advance will also allow you to circumvent some of these issues (see Chapter 8), allowing you to tailor the training to genuinely meet the needs of the trainees. Finally, it is worth stating that not everyone is an ideal candidate for communication skills training. Candidacy is a fascinating concept and there is little research examining candidacy for speech and language therapy interventions overall. Not everyone is receptive to change. Not everyone is ready for change. Not everyone is cognitively able to change. But SLTs have an important and valuable role to play in improving accessibility and realizing the rights of people with communication difficulties to participate in decision making by reducing as many barriers as possible.

Some of the content of this chapter is based on independent research arising from a Doctoral Research Fellowship, Anna Volkmer DRF-2015-08-182, supported by the National Institute for Health Research. The views expressed in this publication are those of the author and not necessarily those of the NHS, the National Institute for Health Research or the Department of Health.

References

Allen, J. & Marshall, C.R. (2015). Parent–Child Interaction Therapy (PCIT) in school-aged children with specific language impairment. *International Journal of Language & Communication Disorders*, 1-14.

Allwood, R., Pilnick, A., O'Brien, R., Goldberg, S., Harwood, R.H., & Beeke, S. (2017). Should I stay or should I go? How healthcare professionals close encounters with people with dementia in the acute hospital setting. *Social Science & Medicine, 191*, 212-225.

Beeke, S., Sirman, N., Beckley, F., Maxim, J., Edwards, S., Swinburn, K., & Best, W. (2013). *Better Conversations with Aphasia: An e-learning resource*. Available at: https://extend.ucl.ac.uk/

Beeke, S., Johnson, F., Beckley, F., Heilemann, C., Edwards, S., Maxim, J., & Best, W. (2014). Enabling better conversations between a man with aphasia and his conversation partner: Incorporating writing into turn taking. *Research on Language and Social Interaction, 47*(3), 292–305. DOI: 10.1080/08351813.2014.925667

Beeke, S., Beckley, F., Johnson, F., Heilemann, C., Edwards, S., Maxim, J., & Best, W. (2015) Conversation focused aphasia therapy: Investigating the adoption of strategies by people with agrammatism. *Aphasiology, 29*(3), 355–377 DOI:10.1080/02687038.2014.881459.

Best, W., Beckley, F., Edwards, S., Heilemann, C., Howard, D., Johnson, F., Maxim, J., & Beeke, S. (2016). Conversation therapy with people with aphasia and conversation partners using video feedback: A group and case series investigation of changes in interaction. *Frontiers in Human Neuroscience, 10*, 562.

Blom Johansson, M., Carlsson, M., Ostberg, P., & Sonnan-Der, K. (2013). A multiple-case study of a family-oriented intervention practice in the early rehabilitation phase of persons with aphasia. *Aphasiology, 27*, 201–226.

Carling-Rowland, A., Black, S., McDonald, L., & Kagan, A. (2014). Increasing access to fair capacity evaluation for discharge decision-making for people with aphasia: A randomized controlled trial. *Aphasiology, 28*(6), 750–765.

Craig, P. & Petticrew, M. (2013). Developing and evaluating complex interventions: Reflections on the 2008 MRC guidance. *International Journal of Nursing Studies, 50*(5), 585-587.

Eggenberger, E., Heimerl, K., & Bennett, M.I. (2013). Communication skills training in dementia care: A systematic review of effectiveness, training content, and didactic methods in different care settings. *International Psychogeriatrics, 25*(3), 345-358.

Epstein, R.M., Duberstein, P.R., Fenton, J.J., Fiscella, K., Hoerger, M., Tancredi, D.J., ... & Kaesberg, P. (2017). Effect of a patient-centred communication intervention on oncologist-patient communication, quality of life, and health care utilization in advanced cancer: The VOICE randomized clinical trial. *JAMA Oncology, 3*(1), 92-100.

Forsgren, E., Hartelius, L., & Saldert, C. (2017). Improving medical students' knowledge and skill in communicating with people with acquired communication disorders. *International Journal of Speech-Language Pathology, 19*(6), 541-550.

Heard, R., O'Halloran, R., & McKinley, K. (2017). Communication partner training for health care professionals in an inpatient rehabilitation setting: A parallel randomised trial. *International Journal of Speech-Language Pathology*, 19(3), 277-286.

Hopper, T., Holland, A., & Rewega, M. (2002). Conversational coaching: Treatment outcomes and future directions. *Aphasiology*, 16, 745-761.

Kagan, A. (1998) Supported conversation for adults with aphasia: Methods and resources for training conversation partners. *Aphasiology*, 12(9), 816-830.

Kagan, A., Black, S.E., Duchan, J.F., Simmons-Mackie, N., & Square, P. (2001). Training volunteers as conversation partners using supported conversation for adults with aphasia (SCA): A controlled trial. *Journal of Speech, Language, and Hearing Research*, 44(3), 624-638.

Kruser, J.M., Taylor, L.J., Campbell, T.C., Zelenski, A., Johnson, S.K., Nabozny, M.J., ... & Schwarze, M.L. (2017). "Best case/worst case": Training surgeons to use a novel communication tool for high-risk acute surgical problems. *Journal of Pain and Symptom Management*, 53(4), 711-719.

Lanzi, A., Burshnic, V., & Bourgeois, M.S. (2017). Person-centred memory and communication strategies for adults with dementia. *Topics in Language Disorders*, 37(4), 361-374.

Lock, S., Wilkinson, R., & Bryan, K. (2008). *Supporting Partners of People with Aphasia in Relationships and Conversation*. Milton Keynes: Speechmark.

McCormick, M., Bose, A., & Marinis, T. (2017). Decision-making capacity in aphasia: SLT's contribution in England. *Aphasiology*, 31(11), 1344-1358.

Murphy, J. & Oliver, T. (2013). The use of Talking Mats to support people with dementia and their carers to make decisions together. *Health & Social Care in the Community*, 21(2), 171-180.

Ontario Ministry of Health and Long-Term Care. (1997). *Capacity to Make Admissions Decisions Questionnaire*. http://www.health.gov.on.ca/english/providers/pub/manuals/ccac/cspm_sec_4/4-9.html

Ripich, D.N. (1994). Functional communication with AD patients: A caregiver training program. *Alzheimer Disease and Associated Disorders*, 8, 95-109.

Ripich, D., Ziol, E., & Lee, M.M. (1998). Longitudinal effects of communication training on caregivers of persons with Alzheimer's disease. *Clinical Gerentologist*, 19(2), 37-55.

Ripich, D., Ziol, E., Fritsch, T., & Durand, E.J. (1999). Training Alzheimer's disease caregivers for successful communication. *Clinical Gerentologist*, 21(1), 37-56.

Royal College of Speech and Language Therapy (RCSLT) (2014). *SLT Provision for People with Dementia: RCSLT Position Paper*. http://www.rcslt.org/members/publications/publications2/dementia_position_paper2014

Saldert, C., Backman, E., &Hartelius, L. (2013). Conversation partner training with spouses of persons with aphasia: A pilot study using a protocol to trace relevant characteristics. *Aphasiology*, 27, 271-292.

Saldert, C., Forsgren, E., & Hartelius, L. (2016). Teaching medical students about communication in speech-language disorders: Effects of a lecture and a workshop. *International Journal of Speech-Language Pathology, 18*(6), 571-579.

Samsi, K. & Manthorpe, J. (2011). 'I live for today': A qualitative study investigating older people's attitudes to advance planning. *Health & Social Care in the Community, 19*(1), 52-59.

Simmons-Mackie, N.N., Kagan, A., O'Neill Christie, C., Huijbregts, M., McEwen, S., & Willems, J. (2007). Communicative access and decision making for people with aphasia: Implementing sustainable healthcare systems change. *Aphasiology, 21*(1), 39-66.

Simmons-Mackie, N., Savage, M.C., & Worrall, L. (2014). Conversation therapy for aphasia: A qualitative review of the literature. *International Journal of Language & Communication Disorders, 49*(5), 511-526.

Small, J.A. & Gutman, G. (2002). Recommended and reported use of communication strategies in Alzheimer caregiving. *Alzheimer Disease and Associated Disorders, 16*(4), 270-278.

Volkmer, A. (2016). *Dealing with Capacity and Other Legal Issues with Adults with Acquired Neurological Conditions: A Resource for Speech and Language Therapists.* Guildford: J&R Press.

Volkmer, A., Spector, A., & Beeke, S. (2018.) Better Conversations with Primary Progressive Aphasia (BCPPA): Asking people with PPA and their families how speech and language therapists could support them to live well and maintain relationships. *Aphasiology,* 1464-5041

Volkmer, A., Spector, A., Warren, J., & Beeke, S. (forthcoming 2019). UK-wide survey of Speech and Language Therapy Practice with people with PPA.

Volkmer, A., Warren, J., Spector, A., & Beeke, S. (In press). The 'Better Conversations with Primary Progressive Aphasia (BCPPA)' program for people with PPA (Primary Progressive Aphasia): Protocol for a randomised controlled pilot study. *Pilot and Feasibility Studies.*

Wilkinson, R., Lock, S., Bryan, K., & Sage, K. (2011). Interaction-focused intervention for acquired language disorders: Facilitating mutual adaptation in couples where one partner has aphasia. *International Journal of Language and Communication Disorders, 13,* 74-87.

6 Supporting multidisciplinary colleagues to develop and use accessible written information materials during capacity assessments

Mark Jayes

Introduction

The legal framework for mental capacity assessment within each of the UK nations requires professionals to provide practical support to help individuals to make decisions, before it can be concluded that they lack capacity. The frameworks recommend that professionals should make available and encourage the use of alternative communication methods to support people with communication difficulties to understand information about decisions and to express their preferences and wishes during mental capacity assessments. These methods should be tailored to support individual needs in order to facilitate both understanding and expression. Chapter 3 of the MCA 2005 Code of Practice (2007) and a guidance document (Scottish Government, 2008) relating to the Adults with Incapacity (Scotland) Act 2000 provide useful information about these issues. In Northern Ireland, Speech and Language Therapists (SLTs) have been consulted about the type of guidance that should be included in the Code of Practice to aid implementation of the new Mental Capacity Act (2016).

As SLTs, we are experts in *inclusive communication*, the use of diverse approaches to support people to understand information and express themselves; these approaches include *total communication, augmentative and alternative communication (AAC)* and *accessible information* methods. We are skilled and experienced in adapting our own communication and in creating novel information materials to support the people we work with to communicate more easily and effectively.

Our expertise in inclusive communication approaches can help us to become better mental capacity *assessors*. We also have a key role to play as *facilitators* of communication between professionals and service users, in

1. Make a case for communication access

⇩

2. Explain inclusive communication

⇩

3. Explain who benefits from accessible information

⇩

4. Explain different approaches to making accessible information

⇩

5. Provide examples of accessible information

⇩

6. Provide a health warning

⇩

7. Explain how to prepare ready-made materials

⇩

8. Explain how to prepare materials for individuals

Figure 6.1 Step-by-step approach to supporting other professionals to develop accessible information.

instances when our multidisciplinary colleagues are the *assessors* or *decision-makers* during capacity assessments. However, another important contribution we can make is as *educators and trainers* in topics related to communication. We have a responsibility to share our inclusive communication knowledge and skills with our colleagues, in order to support them to improve their practice.

This chapter provides guidance and practical tools to help SLTs to support other professionals to provide accessible written information materials during mental capacity assessments. It is designed to provide a step-by-step approach to supporting our multidisciplinary colleagues to recognise the importance of communication access and to understand simple approaches to preparing and trialling accessible information. The content of this chapter could be adapted to form the basis for a training package. The steps involved in this approach are summarised in Figure 6.1 and described in more detail in the following sections.

1. Make a case for communication access

Professionals need to understand the rationale for providing information about decisions in different ways, in order to support people's understanding

Table 6.1 Summary of UK legal requirements to support communication during capacity assessments.

Jurisdiction	Legislation	Requirement
England and Wales	Mental Capacity Act (2005)	Information must be provided "in a way that is appropriate to (the service user's) circumstances" (para 3(2)) "Information must be tailored to an individual's needs and abilities. It must also be in the easiest and most appropriate form of communication for the person concerned" (Department of Constitutional Affairs, 2007, p.31).
Northern Ireland	Northern Ireland Mental Capacity Act (2016)	"For the purposes of providing the information or explanation... in a way appropriate to the person's circumstances it may, in particular, be appropriate (a) to use simple language or visual aids; or (b) to provide support for the purposes of communicating the information or explanation" (para 5(4)).
Scotland	Adults with Incapacity (Scotland) Act 2000	"The present and past wishes and feelings of the adult so far as they can be ascertained by any means of communication, whether human or by mechanical aid (whether of an interpretative nature or otherwise) appropriate to the adult" (para 1 (4)).

so that they can participate in decision making. A good way to approach this is to remind professionals of the requirements of the legal mental capacity framework that applies where they work. As described in the introduction to this chapter, each legislative framework in the UK includes clear requirements for assessors to provide information in formats that support individuals to understand, think about and make decisions. Table 6.1 provides a summary of how each framework articulates this.

Table 6.2 UK legislation and professional standards promoting the use of accessible information.

Jurisdiction	Law/Standard	Link to communication access
UK	UN Convention on the Rights of People with Disabilities (2006)	Accessible information should be provided to all people who require it.
	Equality Act (2010)	It is unlawful to discriminate against people with a communication disability by not providing communication access.
England and Wales	Care Act (2014)	Local authorities have a responsibility to provide accessible information about care and support for adult service users and carers.
England	Accessible Information Standard (2015)	Adult health and social care providers must ask service users about their communication support needs and provide that support.
Northern Ireland	Disability Discrimination Act (1995)	Service providers are required to make reasonable adjustments to their services to help people with disabilities to overcome barriers to access.
	Special Educational Needs and Disability (NI) Order 2005	Educational establishments have a duty to make reasonable adjustments to enable people with disabilities to have the same access to education as people without disabilities.
Scotland	Adult Support and Protection (Scotland) Act 2007	Any public body or officer must assist and facilitate communication using whatever method is appropriate to an individual's needs.
	Mental Health (Care and Treatment) (Scotland) Act 2003	Agencies should provide information about health care and treatment options in whatever format is required to support an individual with a mental health condition or learning disability to understand it.

It might also be beneficial to remind professionals of other statutory requirements and professional standards relating to accessible information. Table 6.2 summarizes legislation and standards that place requirements on professionals in health and social care to provide accessible information in order to ensure equal access to care services. These could be used to provide persuasive evidence of professionals' responsibilities during mental capacity assessments.

Another way to help professionals think about why information should be presented in different ways is to help them to understand on a personal level what it might feel like not to be able to access information. A really persuasive way to do this is to use the simple exercise below.

Exercise to raise professionals' awareness of the need for accessible information

(a) Ask people if they have the mental capacity to make decisions about their own healthcare.

(b) Show them the information below (e.g., on a PowerPoint slide) and ask them what decision they might make or how they might respond if they received the following information (note that this information is in French but could be translated into other languages, depending on the resources you have available).

> Vous trouvez qu'il est difficile à avaler actuellement. Par la suite, vous n'êtes pas capable de manger suffisamment pour vous garder en bonne santé. Nous voudrions mener une petite procédure afin que nous puissions vous nourrir par un tube dans votre estomac. Les risques de cette procédure sont de possibles démangeaisons, des saignements ou une infection.

(c) Ask people for their responses or reactions. Explore how this situation makes them feel. Check whether they still feel they have the mental capacity to make a healthcare decision. Emphasize to them that the fact that they cannot understand the information about the decision should not mean that they lack mental capacity. Presenting the information in a different language should not alter their inherent decision-making abilities. Explain that this is how it might feel to be someone who speaks or reads a different language or has a communication difficulty and is not supported adequately to make a decision.

(d) Provide a translation for the information above (see example below) and explore how people now feel about the information. Ask whether they could make a decision based on this information and what questions they might wish to ask about the procedure.

> You are having difficulties swallowing. As a result, you cannot eat enough to maintain your health. We would like to conduct a small procedure so that we can feed you through a tube into your stomach. The risks of this procedure are possible itching, bleeding or infection.

2. Explain inclusive communication

It is important to help other professionals understand the nature and importance of inclusive communication. Use the RCSLT Inclusive Communication clinical resource web pages to help you to do this (https://www.rcslt.org/cq_live/resources_a_z/inclusive_communication/overview). These web pages will help you think about ways to define and describe inclusive communication. You can find a link to the RCSLT position paper on inclusive communication (RCSLT, 2016) on the web pages. This document uses inclusive communication as an umbrella term to describe all approaches to supporting people to understand information and express themselves, including total communication, augmentative and alternative communication (AAC) methods and accessible information approaches. It may be helpful to explain each of these terms to other professionals to help them understand inclusive communication. The boxes below provide some sample definitions that could be used to explain these terms.

Total communication
The use of any communication method to support an individual to maximize her or his ability to communicate (Rautakoski, 2011). These methods can be verbal (involving speech and language) or nonverbal. They include speech and writing, any type of vocalization, use of images (including line drawings, photographs, symbol systems, cartoons and video), objects and physical actions (including gesture, pointing at things, facial expression and mime). These methods can be used by the individual with the communication difficulty and by those who communicate with her or him.

Augmentative and alternative communication (AAC)
The use of different methods to supplement or replace speech and language (Beukelman & Mirenda, 2005). AAC may include the use of total communication methods (e.g., sign systems, gesture, facial expression). These methods can be used without the need for any type of communication device or aid. Alternatively, AAC can involve communication aids. Aids can be 'low-tech', such as individualized communication books or alphabet charts; they can also be 'high-tech' (e.g., involving speech generating devices or computer software).

Accessible information
Information that is presented in such a way that it can be understood and used easily by its target audience (Litherland, 2007). There are several approaches to adapting information to make it more accessible to people with communication difficulties. What these approaches have in common is that they tend to involve the use of simplified language and different visual adaptations to make text-based information easier to read and understand. These visual adaptations include changes to the text font style and size, changes to text formatting to limit the amount of information presented on a page, and the inclusion of different images alongside the text to support people to understand the most important information.

3. Explain who benefits from accessible information

Professionals who have not received specialist training in communication disorders find it difficult to identify people with communication needs and do not understand how to support their needs. It is helpful when talking to other professionals about accessible information to give an overview of the types of people who may benefit from its provision. This overview should include introductory information about different communication disorders and how these impact on different communicative abilities. It is also beneficial to provide information about the types of medical conditions or labels that are associated with different communication disorders, in order to help our multidisciplinary colleagues to understand better which service users should be offered accessible information materials. Figure 6.2 provides summary information about different communication disorders that could form the basis of a training presentation slide. It might also be beneficial to talk about dysarthria, dysphonia and apraxia of speech and to explain how these disorders do not affect the ability to understand language but may co-occur with aphasia or another disorder affecting use of language.

- **Aphasia**

  Difficulty using language (spoken and written)

  Associated with stroke and some types of dementia

- **Cognitive-communication disorders**

  Impact of cognitive changes on language, social communication

  Associated with brain injury, neurodegenerative conditions (including dementia), mental health conditions

- **Developmental disorders**

  Effects on speech, language, reasoning, social use of language

  Associated with learning disabilities, autistic spectrum disorders

---

Figure 6.2 Sample summary information about communication disorders.

Table 6.3 Guidelines for making written information accessible to different clinical populations.

Clinical population	Producing organization	Name of guidance
People with hearing and visual difficulties	Social Care Institute for Excellence (SCIE)	How to produce information in an accessible way (SCIE, 2005) Available at: http://www.scie.org.uk/
Stroke survivors	Stroke Association	Accessible information Guidelines (Stroke Association, 2012) Available at: https://www.stroke.org.uk/shop/product/accessible-information-guidelines
	National Institute for Health Research (NIHR) Clinical Research Network: Stroke	Engaging with people who have aphasia: a set of resources for stroke researchers (NIHR, 2014). Available at: http://www.crn.nihr.ac.uk/blog/news/new-aphasia-resources-for-researchers-conducting-stroke-studies/
People with intellectual or learning disabilities	Change / National Equality Partnership	How to make information accessible: a guide to producing easy read documents (CHANGE / National Equality Partnership 2009). Available at: http://www.changepeople.org/free-resources/
	Department of Health (DH)	Making written information easier to understand for people with learning disabilities (DH, 2010). Available at: https://www.gov.uk/government/publications/making-written-information-easier-to-understand-for-people-with-learning-disabilities-guidance-for-people-who-commission-or-produce-easy-read-information-revised-edition-2010
	Social Care Institute for Excellence (SCIE)	How to produce information in an accessible way (SCIE, 2005) Available at: http://www.scie.org.uk/
People living with brain injury	Headway	Coping with communication problems after brain injury (Headway, 2014) Available at: https://www.headway.org.uk/shop.aspx
People living with dementia	Dementia Engagement and Empowerment Project (DEEP)	Writing dementia-friendly information (DEEP, 2013) Available at: http://dementiavoices.org.uk/wp-content/uploads/2013/11/DEEP-Guide-Writing-dementia-friendly-information.pdf

4. Explain different approaches to making accessible information

It is important to make people understand that information should be adapted to make it accessible to the target user group. A key message to communicate here is that **one size does not fit all**. Different groups of information users have different needs, depending on the nature of their particular communication disability. For example, people with intellectual or learning disabilities are likely to have different needs to people living with dementia or aphasia.

It is helpful to make professionals aware of a number of guidelines that exist to guide the production of accessible information for people with communication difficulties. These are summarized in Table 6.3.

Ideally, anyone adapting information to make it accessible should make use of guidance that relates to the clinical population they are seeking to target. However, sometimes it is not possible to produce different sets of resources for different groups due to resource restrictions. Although the guidelines do contain slightly different recommendations for adapting information for individual clinical populations, there are number of broad principles that could applied to any clinical group. These are summarized in Figure 6.3. It may be helpful to share these principles directly with other professionals or to use them to plan your own training.

5. Provide examples of accessible information

It is likely that professionals will need to see practical applications of these principles in order to fully understand them. People without a background in linguistics or communication may not understand what "simple, everyday words and sentence structures" look like. It may be helpful to provide clarification about the features of simple language. Figure 6.4 gives some practical guidance about how language can be simplified, based on the guidelines summarized in Table 6.3.

A useful resource to help professionals gauge whether they are using simple language is to use the Flesch-Kincaid (Kincaid et al., 1975) readability function in the proofing options available in Microsoft Word. This function analyzes the complexity of the language in a document, in terms of word and sentence length. It then provides a *grade level* – a numeric score that indicates how easy the document should be to read. The Stroke Association guidelines (2012) for making information accessible to people with aphasia recommend

1. Use simple, everyday words and sentence structures.
2. Use short sentences with one main idea per sentence.
3. Use clear photographs to illustrate important single concepts.
4. Use communication symbols if the reader is familiar with them.
5. Use a sans serif font of at least size 14 point.
6. Highlight important information using bold, headings and text boxes.
7. Break up text using line spacing, bullet points, headings and white space.
8. Involve the target audience in the creation of adapted information.

- **Use plain, everyday** language (but not childish language)
- Avoid jargon and acronyms
- Use short sentences (5–15 words)
- Put only one main idea in each sentence
- Use present tenses
- Use the active voice not passive (you may need to explain this)
- Use personal language, e.g. "we" and "you"

Figure 6.3 Practical guidance about how language can be simplified.

that, ideally, text should have a grade level of 5 or below for it to be accessible to this group.

It is a good idea to have a selection of preprepared materials that you can use to illustrate accessible information principles. For example, in relation to the earlier example about swallowing (Section 1), you could show the information in the box below to provide an example of how language has been simplified to support people to understand the text.

We would like to conduct a small procedure so that we can feed you through a tube into your stomach. The risks of this procedure are possible itching, bleeding or infection.

- We can give you food through a small tube.
- We put the tube through a hole into your stomach.
- The hole may itch or bleed.
- You may feel unwell after we put the tube in.

(Similarly, you could use the information below to illustrate how textual information can be formatted and how images can be added to increase its accessibility.)

We can give you **food** through small **tube**.

We put the **tube** through a **hole** in your **stomach**..

Figure 6.4 Common content and design principles for making written information accessible to people with communication disorders.

6. Provide a health warning:
Accessible information is not a panacea

It is essential to emphasize to professionals that use of these population-specific guidelines or the general principles will not guarantee that people with communication disabilities will find the information easier to read or understand more of its content. Due to the nature and severity of their specific communication difficulties people will have individual information needs.

The effectiveness of methods to make information more accessible to people with communication difficulties has not been widely researched. The available evidence does suggest that using these methods to adapt information may help some but not all people with communication disabilities to understand more information. People with milder difficulties are more likely to benefit from adapted information, whereas people with more severe difficulties may not (Jayes & Palmer, 2014). In order to illustrate this point to other professionals, it may be helpful to ask them to think about the fact that some people with mobility difficulties can walk using a stick, whilst others may need a walking frame and yet others may not be able to walk at all and will need to use a wheelchair to mobilize.

It is also important that professionals understand that people with communication disabilities may have specific preferences about the types of information materials they wish to receive; some may not want to use adapted information formats during mental capacity assessments. People with communication difficulties have different views on accessible information; whilst many people appreciate adaptations to information content and design, some may not want to receive this type of information because they could find it patronizing or insulting (Rose et al., 2012). Family carers and friends may also find such materials patronizing. This could mean that some people may be reluctant to use adapted materials, even when these materials may help people with communication difficulties to understand more information.

Furthermore, different cultural, ethnic and religious groups may have particular preferences about the nature of any written information they receive. It is essential that anyone preparing information resources considers the language needs of different groups and also the way that cultural differences may influence the way that information is presented. At the same time, it is always important to remember that individuals within a particular group are likely to have individual preferences and needs. It is not necessarily the responsibility of SLTs to provide training to other professionals about these issues, but it is important that we encourage our colleagues from other disciplines to be aware of them. A good source of information on such issues would be your organization's patient information manager or its equality and diversity lead.

Professionals need to understand that it is always important to trial the information with its target users to check that it is effective and acceptable, before using the materials during mental capacity assessments. Trialling the information with representatives of a particular clinical group will help to establish that these materials actually help people with similar communication needs to communicate more effectively. Practical ways to approach this are discussed below in Section 7.

7. Explain how to prepare ready-made materials

The practical steps below can be used to create ready-made accessible information materials for use with groups of people. You could use these steps when preparing accessible information training materials.

(a) Identify what type of information needs to be included

The first thing to consider for anyone planning to produce adapted information materials is to identify what type of information needs to be included. It is important to remind other professionals that mental capacity assessments need to be time- and decision-specific, which means any accessible information material should include personalized and contextualized content (e.g., a photograph of a service user's home for a capacity assessment relating to a decision about where the person should live on discharge). Therefore, it will be difficult to prepare comprehensive generic written materials in advance that can be used in every capacity assessment. However, it should be possible to prepare some general information about common treatment and care decisions (e.g., common surgical procedures, treatment options or care arrangements) that can used to support the capacity assessment process for many service users.

When preparing these materials, professionals need to ensure they include **relevant information** about the decision the service user is being asked to make. In order to help professionals identify what constitutes relevant information, you should direct them to any guidance documents that support the mental capacity legislation for their nation. Relevant information should always include the following:

- What the decision is

- The reason why the decision is needed now

- The decision options available to the person

- The known benefits and risks associated with each option

- The likely consequences of choosing each option, or of not making any decision at all.

(b) Check if any existing materials could be used

Encourage professionals to check whether suitable materials already exist and could be used locally in their current format or be adapted for local use. A patient information manager or the medical illustration department for the local organization may have a library of existing resources. Alternatively, professionals working in a local organization or further afield may have materials that could be shared. It is important to explore professional networks before devoting considerable resources to creating new information materials, to avoid 'reinventing the wheel'.

(c) Decide which accessible information approach to use

Professionals will need to decide which guidance to follow when creating any novel materials (see Section 4 above). This will largely depend on the target clinical population for whom the resource is being developed. If professionals wish to develop more generic resources to use with diverse groups of service users, it may be appropriate to use the general principles outlined in Figure 6.3. It is important to remind your colleagues that when they create accessible materials for use in mental capacity assessments, they should aim to do what is practicable with the resources available to them. It may not be possible to create perfect resources for use with every service user group. However, they need to be able to demonstrate that they have done as much as possible during a capacity assessment to support an individual's decision-making abilities.

(d) Involve service users in the design process

It is essential that anyone creating novel information materials should ask members of the target user group for the information to be involved in its design. Asking people with communication difficulties to review and provide feedback on accessible information should help to increase the information's effectiveness and also its acceptability to the target group. It is important for professionals to ask these people the following questions about the information:

- Do they think the language is easy to understand?
- Are there any words that they do not understand?
- Is the text easy to read?

- Do they recognize any images used and understand why they have been included?
- Do they like the look of the information?
- Is there too much information on the page?
- Is there anything that they do not like or think should be omitted?
- Is there anything missing?

Involving service users in information design can be challenging and time-consuming and for it to be successful considerable skill and preparation is required. Again, it is important for professionals to recruit support with these aspects of information design from existing resources. The employing organization may have service user involvement panels that include people with communication difficulties; these people may be willing to review information materials and the panel may have a professional facilitator who can support professionals during this review process. The organization's patient information manager or equality and diversity lead should be able to advise if these panels exist locally. Alternatively, it would be worthwhile enquiring whether local or national charities representing people with communication disabilities are able to review materials in person, by post, or electronically. Chapter 7 discusses the involvement of service users in co-production and co-delivery further.

(e) Consider piloting prototype materials

Once professionals have developed a prototype version of any new accessible information resource, they should consider piloting the materials with members of the target recipient group for the information. Ideally, this should take place in the context in which the information is designed to be used, i.e., within mental capacity assessments. This will help to establish if the materials can be used functionally and are 'fit for purpose'.

Professionals should be invited to use the materials during a set number of capacity assessments. These individuals can then be asked about their experience of using the materials and particularly about any difficulties they encountered as they used them. Ideally, service users receiving the information during a capacity assessment should be asked to provide feedback on the materials, in order to assess their effectiveness and acceptability in a real-world context.

After a capacity assessment involving use of the new materials, professionals should attempt to ask service users questions relating to how easy the information was to use and whether it contained acceptable language and images; they should also ask service users whether they think the materials helped them to understand more information about the decision involved in the capacity assessment. It may be beneficial for SLTs to support other professionals in collecting this type of information from service users with communication difficulties.

(f) Revise prototype materials based on feedback

It is essential to use any feedback gathered from the trial period to make changes to the materials. Ideally, the revised materials should then be reviewed by the professionals and service users who suggested changes to the documents, in order to check that the revisions are adequate.

(g) Implement materials within usual practice

At the end of this process, the accessible information materials can be introduced to the wider local professional community for use within mental capacity assessments. It is important that SLTs take a leadership role in explaining to other professional groups how to incorporate the use of accessible information materials during mental capacity assessments. Other professionals need to understand that, in most circumstances, written materials should be used to supplement and not replace spoken explanations during discussions about decision options. It may be that for some individuals in certain service user groups (e.g., people who have hearing impairments), written information alone is sufficient; however, it is likely that most service users with communication difficulties will benefit from being offered accessible written information in conjunction with spoken explanations using simplified language. SLTs can support multidisciplinary colleagues to develop, practise and improve their skills in using simplified spoken language and other communication strategies, through education and training. At the same time, we should encourage colleagues to refer to speech and language therapy for specialist communication support during capacity assessments, if they feel this is required.

Other professionals also need to be reminded that some service users may not wish to receive adapted information materials and that the use of such materials will not guarantee that all service users who receive them will understand the information contained within them. Finally, it is important to note that like any novel document, accessible information materials should always be reviewed at regular intervals to check that they contain accurate information in the most effective format to be both useful and usable.

The case studies presented on the RCSLT CQ Live Inclusive Communication web pages (https://www.rcslt.org/cq_live/resources_a_z/inclusive_ communication/overview) provide examples of how accessible materials have been developed in different areas of the UK for use with different groups of people with communication difficulties.

8. Explain how to prepare materials for individuals

The practical steps below can be used to create accessible information materials for use with individual service users. You could use these steps when preparing accessible information training materials.

(a) Identify an individual's communication support needs

It is important to explain to our multidisciplinary colleagues that they will need to identify what type of communication support an individual service user needs and wishes to receive, in order to ascertain if accessible information materials may be beneficial to her/him. For example, some service users may experience significant reading difficulties and may find written information too challenging to use; other people may not be able to recognize and derive meaning from visual images sufficiently well to benefit from the inclusion of photographs or pictures in accessible materials. Thus, it is important for professionals to identify any sensory, communication and also cognitive needs that may require support and may influence whether or which form of accessible information is likely to be beneficial.

Perhaps the simplest way to gather this information is to ask the service user, family carers or other people who know the person well what type of support is required or preferred. An important person to approach for information would of course be an SLT or other professional who has worked with the service user previously. It would be important to check what sort of approach has been used before to support the person to think about and make other decisions. Alternatively, this information may be available in the person's care record or in a communication passport. It is important to encourage our colleagues to refer directly to speech and language therapy for a communication assessment in situations where they are unsure about a service user's communication abilities and needs.

(b) Use ready-made information materials

Based on an individual's communication support needs and preferences, it may be possible to use materials that have already been prepared using the process described in Section 7 above. It is important that other professionals realize that it is still essential to check before commencing a capacity assessment that a service user can use the materials functionally and wants to use them during the capacity assessment. It would be useful to introduce the materials to the service user before the capacity assessment to judge how well the individual is able to read the text, recognize any images included in the information, and whether the individual appears happy to use the information. Again, professionals should be encouraged to seek assistance from an SLT if they are unsure whether an individual will be able to use materials.

(c) Create bespoke information materials

In the absence of any existing resource that meets an individual's communication needs and preferences, it will be necessary to create novel materials. The iterative process previously described in Section 7 can be used to create bespoke materials. Again, it is important to emphasize to our colleagues that they should seek our guidance and practical assistance if they require help to develop these materials.

When working with other professionals, we should encourage them to recognize that they may already have the necessary skills to communicate with people who have milder speech, language and communication needs during capacity assessments. When other professionals are enabled to use both spoken and written communication strategies during mental capacity assessments, they may not need to refer to speech and language therapy for specialist support in every case. However, it is important that we also help professionals to recognize in which situations they should seek support from SLTs. Any mental capacity assessment involving a person with more severe communication needs should be supported by an SLT. SLTs have expertise in communication assessment and facilitation that can be used to support people to maximize their communicative abilities during the decision-making process.

Conclusion

All professionals working with people with communication disabilities have a responsibility to support these people to express themselves and participate in decision-making. This is particularly true during the process of mental capacity assessment. A way to facilitate communication access during mental capacity assessments is to provide accessible information materials that relate to different decisions service users are asked to make. As SLTs, we can play a key role in supporting our multidisciplinary colleagues to prepare and use accessible information capacity assessments. This chapter has provided practical suggestions for how SLTs might approach discussions with other professionals about accessible information. Its content can be used as a basis for planning training for other professionals on this topic.

This chapter is based on independent research arising from a Clinical Doctoral Research Fellowship supported by the National Institute for Health Research (NIHR) and Health Education England (HEE).

Any views expressed in this chapter are those of the author and not necessarily those of the NHS, the NIHR, the HEE or the Department of Health.

References

Beukelman, D.R. & Mirenda P. (2005). *Augmentative and Alternative Communication: Supporting Children and Adults with Complex Communication Needs*, 3rd ed. Baltimore MA: Paul H. Brookes Publishing Co.

Department of Constitutional Affairs (2007). *Mental Capacity Act Code of Practice*. London: Department of Constitutional Affairs.

Jayes, M. & Palmer, R. (2014). Initial evaluation of the Consent Support Tool: A structured procedure to facilitate the inclusion and engagement of people with aphasia in the informed consent process. *International Journal of Speech-Language Pathology*, 16(2), 159–168.

Kincaid, J.P. et al. (1975). Derivation of New Readability Formulas (Automated Readability Index, Fog Count, and Flesch Reading Ease formula) for Navy Enlisted Personnel. Research Branch Report 8-75. Chief of Naval Technical Training: Naval Air Station Memphis. Available from: http://digitalcollections.net.ucf.edu/cdm/ref/collection/IST/id/26253

Litherland, R. (2007). Developing the resources people with dementia need. *Journal of Dementia Care*, 15(6), 15–17.

Royal College of Speech and Language Therapists (2016). *Inclusive Communication and the Role of Speech and Language Therapy*. Royal College of Speech and Language Therapists Position Paper. Available from: https://www.rcslt.org/cq_live/resources_a_z/docs/inclusive/ICposition_paper

NHS England Accessible Information Standard (2015) Available from: https://www.england. nhs.uk/ourwork/patients/accessibleinfo/

Rautakoski, P. (2011). Training total communication. *Aphasiology*, *25*(3), 344–365.

Stroke Association (2012). Accessible Information Guidelines. Available from: https://www. stroke.org.uk/shop/product/accessible-information-guidelines

The Scottish Government (2008). *Adults with Incapacity (Scotland) Act 2000. Communication and Assessing Capacity: A Guide for Social Work and Health Care Staff.* Edinburgh: The Scottish Government. Available from: http://www.gov.scot/ Publications/2008/02/01151101/0

7 Service user involvement in MCA and communication training

Anna Volkmer

Introduction

Speech and language therapists (SLTs) are trained to deliver person-centred interventions. When setting goals for therapy an SLT prioritizes the views of the person they are working with, they endeavour to plan interventions that are useful and meaningful to service users' lives. In fact, this type of 'buy in' improves therapeutic outcomes. With these principles of person-centred practice in mind, involving service users in planning and delivering broader aspects of the services we provide seems totally logical. "Utilizing individuals' knowledge and experiences of conditions for the benefit of others is a particular strength of user involvement" (Mockford, Staniszewska, Griffiths, & Herron-Marx, 2011, p. 36).

In 1997, the Department of Health published a White Paper on greater involvement of the public, patients and carers in decision making about local National Health Services (NHS). Yet Patient and Public Involvement (PPI) or service user involvement is more important today than ever before. Health research funders such as the National Institute for Health Research (NIHR) require researchers to have implemented PPI in their applications and to have considered building capacity for this into their projects. The Health Research Authority for NHS England considers this a valuable addition to ethical applications for health care research. The National Institute for Care in Excellence (NICE) and Social Care Institute in Excellence (SCIE) make recommendations on service user involvement in their Decision-making and Mental Capacity Guidelines. In fact, these NICE SCIE guidelines state that "where appropriate, training should be interdisciplinary, involve experts by experience..." (NICE SCIE, p. 4). Local and national policies on developing services emphasise the value of this at all levels of health and care.

This chapter defines service user involvement and highlight why we, as SLTs, should consider this when planning training in relation to decision-making capacity. Examples of how this may work in practice are outlined and include ideas on how to reduce barriers for people with communication difficulties to participating in service user involvement discussions. Finally, evaluating the effectiveness of this approach to service design will also be considered with reference to other chapters in this book.

Definition

The concept we are describing is referred to variously as 'involvement of experts by experience', 'patient and public involvement', 'user involvement', 'service user involvement' or 'lay involvement' (Mockford et al., 2011). There is little consensus on how to describe service user involvement. Mockford et al. recently conducted a systematic review of the use of service user involvement in the UK NHS. They report little agreement in how to define service user involvement across the 28 studies they reviewed. They conclude by describing service user involvement as "multifaceted and includes engagement and communication with the local community focused on outcomes and improving local primary care services, based on building strong relationships between users and those in decision-making roles, direct, sustainable involvement at all levels, openness and acceptance and support" (Mockford et al., 2011, p. 35).

As part of Mockford et al.'s (2011) systematic review they examine the studies for reference to any theoretical background for use of service user involvement. Only one of the two examples they found seem relevant to SLT: namely, the theory that through collective self-advocacy (i.e., advocating for the community you are part of) you can bring back the balance of power from those who hold power over the group, e.g., health professionals. Pearl and Cruice (2017) remind us that "aphasia can limit the extent to which an individual appears competent in daily life" (p. 67). This can shift the power balance toward the more 'competent' people: the health and social care professionals. By including people with communication difficulties in service user involvement we can therefore provide opportunities to shift the balance of power away from the health professionals. This reduces the risk of paternalizing service users by focusing on what we believe is the best for them; instead, this model encourages us to work together with service users to develop services that actually meet the needs of the community we work with.

It is important to note that involving service users in research in this way is quite distinct from how they might participate as a subject of research. In service user involvement people advise on a project and might even be employed as co-researchers (NIHR Research Design Service, viewed 2018). INVOLVE is an organization funded by the UK government to support active patient and public involvement in the NHS, public health and social care research. They define this as: work (research or services) designed and delivered 'by' and 'with' rather than 'for' and 'to' service users. This means that research or services are conceived, designed and delivered with service users as members of the 'team'. INVOLVE emphasizes that including service users from the planning stages through to the execution stages of a project is desirable, rather than simply consulting on a one-off basis to check for approval. Although any kind of consultation is useful, this is exactly what it is – consultation rather than co-development.

Why do we need to consider service user involvement?

When designing a product, companies find out what their customers would like through consultation. As consumers, we are used to giving feedback on the services we receive, through feedback forms, surveys, market research and even complaints. As citizens, we vote for those we feel can lead us. As health professionals, we often imagine what might work best for our service users. But we don't live with the same health conditions as our service users

Fudge, Wolfe and McKevitt (2008) have described user involvement as a phenomenon explained by "several philosophical and political perspectives: consumerism, democracy and citizenship, and the rise of patient pressure groups." (Fudge et al., 2008, p. 1). User groups across areas of health such as maternity, mental health and HIV/AIDS care have advocated for their right to be involved in service development (Fudge et al., 2008). Fudge et al. (2008) also report that professionals in their study "believed in a moral and political commitment to the ethos of involvement and belief in the engagement of citizens in public decision making. Other professionals saw involvement as an NHS requirement, tending to involve service users at the end of the process to get approval for a product or service" (Fudge et al., 2008, p. 5).

But what evidence is there that has shown that service users are more likely to identify current and relevant issues? Or that it works? Fudge et al. (2008) conducted an ethnographic review of user involvement in the stroke services within two London-based hospital services. The authors interviewed professionals and service users on what user involvement meant to them, and what the barriers and facilitators were to actually engaging in this activity. They also considered the impact on the service. Interviewees in their study stated that "involving service users ensured that the staff training and patient information materials that were developed were more relevant because they reflected the views of people affected by stroke" (Fudge et al., 2008, p. 4). They also reported that, for service users, involvement resulted in personal gains; "they reported satisfaction in feeling that professionals were listening to them, that their ideas were acted on, and that their experience of stroke was being harnessed to help others." "Throughout the programme service users were observed engaging with the programme for the social opportunities it provided. Service users also described their involvement as helping to increase their knowledge and understanding of stroke." (Fudge et al., 2008, p. 4).

A Cochrane review of consumer involvement found six randomized controlled trials (Nilson et al., 2013) but little evidence of the effect of service user involvement. Still, the review concluded that these studies did demonstrate that service user involvement is feasible and achievable. Nilson et al. (2013) describe the most positive evidence for service user involvement as coming from two trials where service users were involved in writing information materials. The review concluded that "there is moderate quality evidence that consumer consultation prior to developing patient information material probably results in material that is more relevant, readable and understandable to patients" (Nilson et al, 2013, p. 10).

A recent systematic review examined the impact of service user involvement in research on researchers themselves, the users and the wider community (Brett et al., 2014). The researchers identified 65 articles that they were able to include in their study. These researchers found that service users felt empowered and valued and reported increased confidence. In addition, researchers developed a better understanding of the people involved in their research, and were able to gain an insight into how users think and feel.

The authors suggest that this "may have led to greater respect towards the community they were studying" (Brett et al., 2014, p. 390).

What might be the barriers to involving service users with communication difficulties?

There are many barriers to service user involvement in both clinical and research settings. And for people with communication difficulties there may be an additional layer of complexity. It is worth emphasizing that these barriers are owned by both the professionals and the service users (Fudge et al., 2008). To deal with an issue it can be helpful to anticipate and understand the cause of the issue; thus, the following discussion summarizes some of the research there is on this topic.

Health professionals often have little time and face challenging demands (Mockford et al., 2011; Nilson et al., 2013). Moreover, it is not uncommon that an issue may be perceived as something too technical to consult with service users about. This can mean professionals avoid service user involvement altogether or engage in tokenistic involvement. With little experience of working with service users this cycle continues to make it an even more challenging task to change (Mockford et al., 2011). Even though we may want to change the way we work to involve service users more fully the practicalities of service user involvement do need to be considered. Service user involvement can make research projects costlier and they may take longer when service users are involved (Brett et al., 2014; Mockford et al 2011; Nilson et al, 2013).

Service users may lack an understanding about what and how service user involvement works and may arrive with their own agendas for being involved (Fudge et al., 2008; Mockford et al., 2011). They may have biased views on certain health issues, which may threaten the traditional academic impartiality of knowledge development in health research and the delivery of equitable services in healthcare. Service users have generally reported preferring to be involved in short, tangible projects rather than broader more organizational working parties (Fudge et al., 2008). Nilson et al. (2013) report that service users may not find it meaningful to be involved in projects where there are not many opportunities for input and influence.

Just as people with communication difficulties such as aphasia are often excluded from research (Pearl & Cruice, 2017) they are also often excluded from service user involvement activities. Mockford et al. (2014) found that the stroke community has not been as proactive in advocating for service user involvement as other health communities; perhaps due to the age and abilities of people in these groups. This may be similarly applicable for people with communication difficulties such as aphasia, dementia and other progressive neurological conditions.

Training and support may seem like logical methods of reducing some of these barriers, both for professionals and service users. Where service users did not receive adequate training, and support they felt unable to contribute (Brett et al., 2014). There is an even greater risk of this occurring when service users have communication difficulties. The research literature in this area recognizes that representing particular groups in user involvement activities may be more difficult from both an ethical and practical perspective. This would include potentially vulnerable groups such as those with dementia or aphasia. The Public Involvement Impact Assessment Framework Guidance (Popay & Collins, 2014) emphasizes that this does not mean these groups should not be involved but that careful consideration needs to be given to how best to do this.

Barriers to participation in service user involvement are not dissimilar to barriers in day-to-day conversation difficulties for people with communication difficulties. As SLTs we often work on environmental barriers to participation in therapeutic activities. Many of these barriers are considered societal. The barriers are held by the listener, not by the person with communication difficulties. This highlights that these barriers to involvement are a problem for the professionals and researchers themselves (Pearl & Cruice, 2017). Thus, it is they who can and must change their behaviour to address these issues.

That is not to say there are not additional issues – indeed, people with communication difficulties are not a homogenous group. They are all very different, presenting with different severities of communication difficulty and different areas of communication strength. This means that one adaptation to communication will not suit the needs of all service users involved. People with communication difficulties have different styles of communication, just as we do. They have personal preferences that are above and beyond their communication difficulties and areas of strength. An image may mean one thing to one person and quite another to someone else. One person may prefer photos, others line drawings. Adaptations and accessible communication won't make everyone happy.

People with communication difficulties often present with additional needs beyond being able to understand materials they are presented with.

For example, it can be difficult to attend to a group conversation for someone who has delayed processing. Identifying appropriate turns to contribute ideas in a timely manner is challenging. Listening to others for extended periods is tiring and thus consistently engaging over a period of time is also challenging. Cognitive skills such as attention, inhibition and topic maintenance may be part of an individual's overarching impairment. These concurrent difficulties can impact on topic maintenance, balance of turn taking and group dynamics.

People with communication difficulties may have additional physical limitations that may result in accessibility issues. In general, it is more common for people to present with a complex combination of physical and cognitive difficulties. This means ways of accessing meeting rooms, work spaces, writing things down, and using amenities also need to be considered when planning this type of activity. People may have other external limitations that may be resource based; individuals do not always have the time and financial means to spare for these (generally) voluntary roles.

Many of these issues described above can be addressed using the specialist skills of an SLT. As SLTs we have an in-depth and refined understanding of how communication impairments impact upon conversation and participation. We are able to use our clinical skills to reflect on conversation and modify our own behaviour and communication style. This may include using less jargon and terminology, providing written information, using nonverbal skills to seek clarification, and checking that people have understood. Supporting people to express themselves may involve giving them time to expound their opinions, providing alternative means of explaining their ideas and providing a safe environment to contribute, by respecting and valuing what they say. This can be described as supported or inclusive communication.

SLTs can use more creative and innovative approaches both within a session, before and afterwards. Planning and executing activities that allow people to contribute their ideas may require more time and lateral thinking than supporting individual conversations. This planning may be necessary to maximize engagement. Table 7.1 provides an overview of useful reflections that may allow you to engage people as fully as possible.

What does service user involvement look like?

A first step in getting started is thinking through the actual practicalities and what exactly you might do with service users. An important point to start on is that service user involvement does not require ethical approval. This is a big

Table 7.1 An overview of ideas to support people with communication difficulties to participate as service users. This list is not exhaustive – in fact, generating ideas on how to run the group may be best planned by the service users themselves. As individuals or a group, they may have a preference, or a creative and valuable idea.

Area of consideration	Potential solutions
Setting	Typically, we talk about service user involvement being a group event, where people come together in one room to share ideas on a project. It may be that this is not always feasible and some people may not be able to physically travel anywhere themselves. In this case holding group discussions via video-chat can be helpful. Online mediums can provide a great place for discussion via online chat forums or social media groups if participants are able to engage in this way.
	Engaging people individually is also useful; people may be more honest and engaged. Individualized discussions may also be easier for people with communication difficulties. One-off meetings – visiting people where they are, telephone calls, video calls or email – are all methods of communicating with service users. Even when running group meetings, or holding a separate steering group, it is useful to consider alternative opinions and thus seeking out both group and individual discussions will be useful. The more opinions the better (within what is practical and feasible).
Participants	Inviting people with communication difficulties to participate in service user consultation activities is the most important starting point to involving them. Consider your method of invitation: making contact by phone, advertising at a support group (doing a presentation) or sending clear (aphasia-friendly) invitations.
	Inviting partners, friends or family members of people with communication difficulties to participate alongside the person themselves can be a useful method of maximizing a person's communication. They can prepare a person in advance by presenting and pre-discussing materials or ideas; they can also support a person afterwards to reflect and follow-up on any areas they may have missed (particularly if it was a group meeting).
	Partners, friends or family members may have skills in facilitating an individual's communication and scaffolding their conversation to enable them to participate in a group.
	Partners, friends or family members share the lives of the person with communication difficulties and may have their own unique contributions to make. Respecting all perspectives and ideas can be valuable for service user involvement.
Planning	Liaising with people in advance of an individual meeting or a group meeting can be extremely helpful for both them and you. This type of conversation provides preparation time. Many people may find it easier to plan what they are going to say if they know what the meeting will entail. Informing someone of the content in advance can also ensure they spend less cognitive resources on understanding and more on engaging and contributing. It can also be helpful to have heard some of their ideas in advance in order to build rapport and demonstrate how much you value their contributions by presenting them to the rest of the group (by mutual agreement prior to the meeting).

	This can also allow the group to build on an example or an idea in a truly collaborative way rather than simply approving something you present. Providing people with content and materials in advance of a meeting doesn't need to be this individualized – sending out an agenda (written or image based), sending them materials, a website or a video can be helpful ways of engaging groups.
	It can also be helpful to ask people to do something in advance such as collecting information on a topic to bring to the meeting, perhaps in the form of photos, pictures, objects or written lists. One example of this is where we (the author) asked people to document all their conversation topics (using photos or a written list) over two days and this information was used to brainstorm a hand-out for a therapy session.
	On another more practical note, planning a meeting in terms of exactly what will happen is extremely useful. Sending out an agenda makes people feel valued and respected. Presenting information (for example using flip charts, white boards, power point or video) provides structure and enables you to employ a variety of visual and interactive materials. Prepare these in advance – make sure you have the post-it notes, materials (using creative materials can include counters for voting, cards) (see image above): Lego (for building or counting), playdough (creative expression), pens (drawing/writing) for your chosen activities.
Visual/written materials	Using visual aids is always useful when working with people with communication difficulties. This includes a written and pictorial agenda and minutes. Using the images created by Pearl and Cruice (2017) is helpful.
	Whiteboards, flip charts, paper-based materials are all helpful. Try to consider how people can contribute without having to explain something verbally – perhaps voting, bringing materials (photos/letters/other information) to contribute to a visual brainstorm, using images to convey meanings.
The language you use	You may decide to co-chair a meeting or rotate the chair role within the group. Whatever you do ensure that the language you use demonstrates the utmost respect for the service users. When talking with people use a collective term, e.g., us, our project – avoiding phrases like 'them' and 'you' and not describing it as 'my project'. If you have a meeting with a mixed group (e.g., service users, families and other professionals) start by consulting the service users first. Create a space for people with communication difficulties to contribute and demonstrate that you will all wait for their ideas – they are the most valued.
Documenting the meeting	It can be incredibly useful to take minutes during the meeting or ask someone else to do this (an administrator/student/colleague). This means that you can focus on facilitating the meeting and not having to remember the content. There are other means of documenting the meeting as it occurs, for example taking photos of written plans (whiteboards/flip charts). It can also be helpful to video record or audio record a meeting for later documentation. You do not need to seek ethical approval for this, but you will need to ask for written consent from the participants. For transparency, it may be useful to clearly document when these recordings will be deleted and where they will be stored.

difference between research and service user involvement. In research, you do need ethical approval as you will be using information about, or collected from, participants. In service user involvement people are working with you, collaborating and offering advice – they are not the subjects of research. Having said this, you do need to make sure that people consent to being involved. If you introduce audio and video recording to your activities you will need to be more thorough in gathering documented or written consent for these activities. Your local Trust may have specific guidelines on consent for these activities and it is recommended you check these details against local policy within your organization.

To include service users in your work you need to develop links with them. These links can be made through existing structures; your clinics, third sector organizations, the local community (through newspapers, community groups or social media). Your own organization may already have a list of individuals who are interested and prepared to be involved in service development. In fact, your organization may have support and services available who can advise you extensively on how to do this. Your organization may even have a policy in place. What they may not have are links with people with communication difficulties, nor knowledge of how to overcome some of the barriers of working with people with communication difficulties.

Once you have made contact with service users who have agreed to become involved with your work you can actually involve them. Nilsen et al. (2013) have described the degree of involvement in terms of three tiers: 1. Consultation; asking consumers their views; 2. Collaboration; an active ongoing partnership; 3. Consumer controlled research/activity: with consumers designing, conducting and disseminating information. They advise that service user involvement may be done on an individual basis or by groups of consumers (such as one-to-one interviews, focus groups, citizens' juries, town meetings, committee meetings, working groups) and may use different methods to finalize decisions (such as informal committee consensus, voting, ranking, scoring, visual scales and Delphi surveys).

Other researchers have described categories of service involvement in healthcare in terms of the types of decisions, ideas and changes that were made. Mockford et al. (2011) identified seven categories where service users have influenced health services including: 1. The design and development of buildings and building interiors; 2. Location of services and issues such as parking that might affect the outcome; 3. Development of new services such as evening clinics; 4. Changes to current services such as modifications to the way appointments are arranged; 5. Communication between staff and service users such as co-producing communication standards; 6. Communication between service users such as setting up support groups and 7. Organization of acute trusts such as improvements in hygiene and cleaning services. The authors also report on how service user involvement can directly impact on information development and dissemination and training. It can, for example, influence the development of information leaflets and booklets; raising awareness in the community; and developing and delivering training sessions for professionals around communication.

What you actually do with your service users may depend on where you are working and who you are working with. Fudge et al. (2008) describe a service user involvement project across the stroke services in two London hospitals. People were recruited by sending invitations to individuals on a community stroke register, in local voluntary groups, and to hospital and community clinicians. They held a series of initial meetings to ask service users where they felt stroke services should be improved. Service users were then invited to participate in working groups across these areas. Service users were offered training before they participated in some streams – this included information on how those services worked, the NHS background to the service, and any additional skills that were felt to be useful. Staff were also offered training in supporting services users.

Fudge et al. (2008) describe a range of activities where service users were involved; more actively in some and more passively in others. Active involvement included setting up working groups that planned awareness events at GP surgeries and delivered joint training sessions for other professionals. Service users produced a service user handbook, picture menus in stroke units, information leaflets about parenting after a stroke and distributed these at the awareness events. They also worked on a good practice guide and an accompanying DVD of service users' experiences that was produced and used in staff training sessions. These training sessions focused on educating staff on what it is like having a stroke and how service users wish to be cared for. Passive user involvement was described as "patient satisfaction surveys and suggestion boxes or consultation with service users in the later stages of a project" (Fudge et al., 2008, p. 5).

The NIHR provide specific guidance on involving service users and the public in health and social care research (NIHR https:// www.crn.nihr. ac.uk/wp-content/uploads/ mentalhealth/UserCarerResearcherGuidelines May2014_FINAL.pdf and INVOLVE http:// www.invo.org.uk). They provide an overview of how service users and the public can be involved at all stages of the research cycle; prioritization and conception of research ideas, applications for funding, analysis of data, dissemination of information and review and re-prioritization. What this guidance does not do is specifically address how to involve people with communication difficulties in research.

How can people with communication difficulties be involved?

There are very few examples of service user involvement with people with communication difficulties in the research or academic literature. There is, however, some useful research evidence around what people with aphasia prefer. As mentioned, the key difference between research and service user involvement is that when service users are involved as research subjects the research is 'done to' them, whilst when they are involved as service users they are 'doing' the research 'with you'. In aphasia research, you would ideally include people in both roles – both in planning and doing the research and as participants. The people who are involved as service users cannot also be research participants, because they are like you – they are part of the investigatory/development team and they may bias the work. Similarly, ideally you wouldn't involve service users in planning a service if they were currently using the service. You would invite them as previous service users or service users by (past) experience. To include service users in developing a project you do not need to apply for ethical approval, but to include them as research participants you do. Should you wish to use a quote, a photo or develop materials with your service users you would, however, need to gain appropriate consent to use these images.

Rose et al. (2011) conducted a research study where they gathered information, through semi-structured interviews, on how people with aphasia preferred educational materials about stroke and aphasia to be presented. This study used qualitative research methods to analyze results. This was a research study and participants were involved as research subjects, However, the information collected is incredibly useful and can be used to guide development of educational materials. Data collected included a preference for san serif font, bolding and italicizing of words to highlight key information, bulleting of key points, use of colour, and language conveyed with short words, phrases, sentences, and paragraphs (Rose et al., 2011).

Pearl and Cruice (2017) provide a comprehensive description of the process of involving people with communication difficulties as a user group in their project. This project was funded by the NIHR to develop accessible resources for researchers to use when gaining consent from people with aphasia. Pearl and Cruice (2017) have written a detailed description of the process they went through in this article: providing an overview of the exact format they used to conduct meetings, identifying priorities for the project and methods of achieving the tasks for the project. The researchers describe how they recruited people with aphasia and a carer from a support group they ran (at Speakability). They had a very short period of time to complete the project and decided to recruit users who had some understanding of the role they were being asked to participate in. They held 14 meetings between three and four hours long, with appropriately scheduled rest and refreshment breaks. Chairing and time keeping of meetings was shared by service users and the project leaders. Pearl and Cruice (2017) describe how they established an ethos of respect by valuing one another equally as experts. The meetings focused on identifying preferences for resources and developing images and text for the resource. Service users worked with designers to help them understand the needs of people with aphasia, co-design ideas and act as models for the images. These were then reviewed and modified to meet the needs and expectations of the group. In this process, a set of key principles were agreed such as colour coding and style.

Once reviewed and agreed the group developed sample templates of how the resources should be used by researchers in practice. The added value of including service users in this project is clear. The materials developed in this project have consequently been published on the NIHR website and are freely available for use at https://www.nihr.ac.uk/nihr-in-your-area/stroke/aphasia. htm. Pearl and Cruice (2017) finish the article with recommendations for future research in the area of inclusion, accessible information and the SLT role in gaining consent for research.

There are some other examples of service user involvement with people with communication difficulties including dementia (primary progressive aphasia) and people who use communication aids to communicate that can be found on other mediums including social media. The author's (Volkmer, 2017 blog entry) own research blog includes descriptions of engaging service users in a steering committee which oversees and advises on a current research project: https://annavolkmersbigphdadventure.wordpress.com/2017/11/13/ engaging-the-experts-in-every-which-way/. The steering committee for this project are meeting three times annually throughout the four years of the project. The steering committee is made up of three couples where each couple includes a person with Primary Progressive Aphasia (PPA). Alongside these couples are professionals including a nurse specialist, an SLT from a third sector organization and a neuropsychologist. These people were recruited through the researcher's links with support group organizations (advertising at their meetings) and through links with interested service users who had been involved with the original funding application, as well as professional links. Their role was agreed at the first meeting where the ground rules were discussed and agreed: to provide advice on the research project and co-produce materials for the study. The work carried out in the steering groups has included working on participant information forms, consent forms and the development of handouts and materials for an intervention. To support this process the group have engaged in creative methods of including all group members. Some barriers are particular to this group; people with PPA are often diagnosed in their 50s and 60s and some group members continue to work. Technology has allowed some of these group members to participate in meetings via telephone or video conferencing. Other barriers are more specifically related to cognition and communication difficulties. Including some consistent features in the meetings has been useful. For example; an agenda and previous minutes are sent out prior to every meeting using the

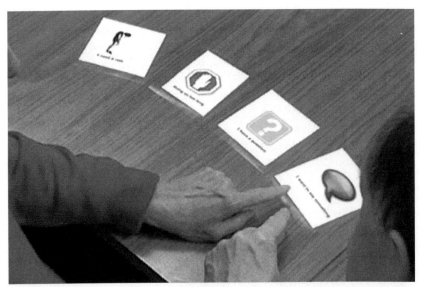

Figure 7.1 Communication cards designed to support group members (from left to right: I need a rest, Going on too long, I have a question, I want to say something)

same aphasia friendly format, every meeting commences with name tags, a lunch and an update before work commences. At every meeting attendees are reminded of the communication cards that were introduced and agreed in the first session to support all group members to ask a question, make a comment, ask for clarification or request a break (see Figure 7.1).

Activities are designed with multiple communication modalities in mind, for example using verbal and visual means to represent information and using verbal and nonverbal means of expression. Figure 7.2 illustrates an example of how the group used post-it notes to vote for work priorities for the group.

Another blog by an SLT also describes engaging in service user activities as part of a PhD research project https://unspokenvoicesproject.wordpress.com/ (Broomfield, viewed February 2018). The author describes using a co-design approach to working with service users. This meant the initial meetings for the project focused on how information should be shared with the service user group. The most significant point that arose was the over reliance on written communication. Consequently, the author describes developing more visual resources – namely, an agenda that used predominantly images. In addition, the author created a video of herself reading the minutes of the last meeting

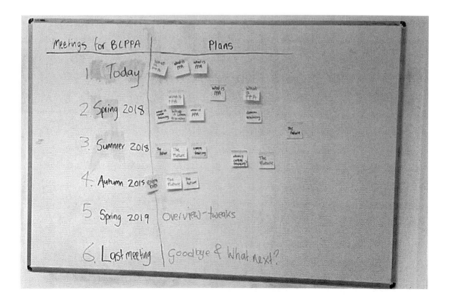

Figure 7.2 Example of using post-it notes to vote for future projects.

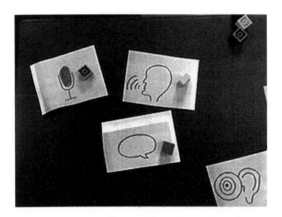

Figure 7.3 Using Lego to vote for a project logo during a service user meeting.

which was sent out on a link to all the group members. Finally she used Lego pieces to vote for preferences during the session (Figure 7.3).

How can we include service user involvement in mental capacity work and training programmes?

At the time of writing the authors are not aware of any examples of service user involvement in mental capacity training in the public domain. Think carefully about the amount of time and resources you have available for this. The less time you have the more you may simply be consulting. In comparison, fully consumer-controlled activities will require a bigger time and resource investment.

Table 7.2 provides some practical ideas of how to involve service users in planning and delivering training around mental capacity. This list is by no means exhaustive. SLTs can think creatively about how they may wish to embed service users into these types of activities. As previously mentioned, the service users themselves may have some equally creative and relevant ideas.

When you are planning and preparing for service user involvement you may wish to consider the group dynamics in more detail. People with progressive diseases may not be able to maintain participation in an activity

Table 7.2 Ideas of how to involve service users in planning and delivering training around mental capacity.

Consultation: Asking service users for their views	Using ongoing collection of feedback forms from service users who have been involved in capacity assessments can be a useful method of gathering information to refine your training materials. You could ask them about their experiences: what therapists, assessors and other staff members did that was or was not helpful. This could provide you with some useful hints and tips, from service users, for professionals you are training.
	You could hold a meeting – a focus group type discussion – before developing the training materials to ask service users what they think should be included. This could also be done on an individual basis by email or telephone, even sending out a questionnaire. You don't need to collect a large volume of information; feedback from one or two people may be useful as a starting point. You could also ask people to share their experiences of being involved in assessments of decision-making capacity in this type of group. These may be useful to include in training materials as direct quotes.
	This type of consultation could continue throughout – developing into a more collaborative piece of work with regular meetings asking for people's views on an ongoing project (see below).
	Developing training materials and holding a one-off meeting afterwards to ask people's opinions is also useful. Be mindful that this isn't simply tokenistic: are you really going to change anything with feedback? Be clear about what can or cannot be changed.
Collaboration: An active ongoing partnership	Collaboration does not require a large group of people. A collaboration may be a partnership with one or two individuals. You could invite people to jointly plan and deliver a presentation with you. The key here is that these materials must be jointly developed, through regular contact and mutual agreement on the training content. This may involve the professional and the service user developing their own sections of a presentation, or the entire training being co-written. Many service users have untapped skills from their current or previous occupations. They may have a strong desire to deliver a presentation or support hands-on training sessions where participants are invited to role-play capacity assessments. This may be a chance for service users to give direct feedback in simulated situations (see Chapter 5 on communication skills training).
	You may wish to establish a regular advisory group or committee who work together to plan the training session with you. This may include aspects of what was described in the previous section (under Consultation) but may be extended so that you use meetings to co-develop handouts for training sessions, create lists of tips and hints, develop a video clip of a capacity assessment that could either depict a 'bad' assessment or a 'good' assessment, or simply record information participants may wish to share. In fact, thinking of the materials in this way is already less of a collaboration and more service user-led. Service users may generate their own innovative ideas about how a training session could be developed or delivered.
	(You may be able to collaborate fully on some aspects of a project and not others – be clear what is and is not up for discussion. You do not need to invite service users to collaborate on every detail.)

(Continued over)

Consumer-controlled research/activity: Consumers designing, conducting and disseminating information	This model may be more challenging for SLTs to facilitate. Consumer-controlled activities might involve a group of service users getting together and planning their own training which they then offer to the service. This might be something an SLT could support a group to do, with an emphasis on the SLT acting as a facilitator, rather than coordinating the project. Service users might take it in turns to coordinate themselves. This type of activity may be most appropriately led by a third sector organization representing the views of service users.

over a longer period, thus you may need to agree a rolling membership as individuals step back. It is important to be clear that, once involved, people may choose to leave at any time. Choosing to include people with progressive and non-progressive communication difficulties in the same group may be tricky. Consider the group milieu: will these particular individuals work well together or could they cause one another distress? How long will your discussion or meeting be? Make sure you are clear on the time requirement, plan regular breaks and consider the time it may take for people to contribute their ideas. Make sure the setting is accessible (are there stairs to climb, are there toilets nearby), that information is provided to cater for different needs and preferences (send letters and email – many people prefer letters) and any other individual issues. The INVOLVE organization provides advice on many of these issues and can act as a useful reference when planning or justifying appropriate costs.

A quick phone call to a previous service user, to ask their opinion on a project, costs less than holding regular meetings where people work together for a number of hours, over a number of months on a single piece of work. Consider this from the perspective of the people you are working with. Service users do not always have the time or the means to be involved. Being involved in a project like this may require them to take time away from work, or caring roles (they may need to employ a carer so they can leave their loved ones at home, they may need to travel some distance). On the other hand, they may be willing to become involved at the expense of other aspects of their lives such as caring for loved ones, attending other social and therapeutic activities and occupational commitments. It is, however, extremely important to consider reimbursing people for their time, work and expenses. Your organization may have a standard policy or method of reimbursing individuals. INVOLVE also provides advice and recommendations about this on their website. They have cost calculators that prompt you to consider and plan costs in advance. This

Table 7.3 Useful resources.

Useful resources
NIHR materials developed for stroke researchers working with people with aphasia (developed by Gill Pearl):
https://www.nihr.ac.uk/nihr-in-your-area/stroke/aphasia.htm.
Inclusive communication guidance from RCSLT:
https://www.rcslt.org/cq_live/resources_a_z/inclusive_communication/resources
INVOLVE specialize in advice on service user involvement, and provide useful materials such as cost calculators, examples of good practice, bursaries for innovative practice:
INVOLVE website: http://www.invo.org.uk/
Specific advice from the National Institute for Health Research on involving service users:
https://www.crn.nihr.ac.uk/wp-content/uploads/mentalhealth/UserCarerResearcherGuidelines May2014_FINAL.pdfandINVOLVE http://www.invo.org.uk

may be useful if you are planning a collaborative piece of work and need to apply for funding. Some basic tips would be to reimburse travel costs and provide adequate refreshments such as food and drinks (make sure you check food preferences in advance). If possible pay people for their time (they are working, after all). This approach to service user involvement demonstrates to them and others that they are a valued, important part of the work. Table 7.3 presents some useful resources to consider in addition to the aforementioned.

Evaluating the impact of service user involvement

Evaluating what we do in clinical practice is second nature. Evaluating service user involvement is also important. The NIHR Research Design Service makes a series of very relevant points on why it can be useful to evaluate service user involvement.

They state that this can help to:

- "identify what works (or not), for whom and in what circumstances

- identify how the involvement impacted on the research process

- celebrate success – recognizing the achievements of your research team and your patients and the public

- generate evidence and share the value of PPI; could your PPI activities inspire others and help evidence the impact of PPI on the research process?

- improve the planning of future projects - evaluating what worked and what didn't will help you identify how to plan future projects."

(NIHR RDS, *Patient and Public Involvement in Health and Social Care Research. A Handbook for Researchers*, p.37).
So how do we evaluate service user involvement? To start, this may be as simple as using a feedback form after a group meeting asking if the setting, refreshments and group activities were adequate and asking for suggestion for forthcoming meetings. Mockford et al.'s (2011) systematic review of the literature in this area reported no validated measurements specifically for capturing the impact of service user involvement. "Data collection was undertaken using questionnaire surveys, semi-structured and structured interviews, focus groups, documentary analysis and observation of meetings. This captured mostly description of the activity and opinion about the difference user involvement has made" (Mockford et al., 2011, p. 35).

Conclusion

Service user involvement is not a novel initiative in the NHS, yet service user involvement is not commonly undertaken with people with communication difficulties. Communication difficulties can present another barrier to service user involvement. However, as SLTs we have a unique set of skills that means we can reduce these barriers.

Service user involvement can be quite liberating in some ways; we do not require ethical approval, we can invite service users from any forum and we can be creative in the ways we work with them. More importantly, service users can make valuable contributions to the training we deliver. In fact, involving service users will provide credence to training. Issues around decision making and mental capacity may be difficult and different for SLTs and other health professionals but service users rely on us to support them at these times. We can learn from their experiences and find out what actually works best; they are the experts by experience.

Some of the content of this chapter is based on independent research arising from a Doctoral Research Fellowship, Anna Volkmer DRF-2015-08-182, supported by the National Institute for Health Research. The views expressed in this publication are those of the author and not necessarily those of the NHS, the National Institute for Health Research or the Department of Health

References

Brett, J., Staniszewska, S., Mockford, C., Herron-Marx, S., Hughes, J., Tysall, C., & Suleman, R. (2014). A systematic review of the impact of patient and public involvement on service users, researchers and communities. *The Patient-Patient-Centered Outcomes Research, 7*(4), 387–395.

Broomfield, K. (blog viewed February 2018). https://unspokenvoicesproject.wordpress.com/

Department of Health (1997). *The New NHS. Modern. Dependable.* London: The Stationery Office.

Fudge, N., Wolfe, C.D., & McKevitt, C. (2008). Assessing the promise of user involvement in health service development: Ethnographic study. *Bmj, 336*(7639), 313–317.

Mockford, C., Staniszewska, S., Griffiths, F., & Herron-Marx, S. (2011) The impact of patient and public involvement on UK NHS health care: A systematic review. *International Journal for Quality in Health Care, 24*(1), 28–38.

NIHR Research Design Service. *Patient and Public Involvement in Health and Social Care Research. A Handbook for Researchers.* Downloaded January 2018 from https://www.nihr.ac.uk/patients-and-public/

Nilsen, E.S., Myrhaug, H.T., Johansen, M., Oliver, S., & Oxman, A.D. (2006). Methods of consumer involvement in developing healthcare policy and research, clinical practice guidelines and patient information material. *Cochrane Database Syst Rev, 3*(3).

Pearl, G. & Cruice, M. (2017). Facilitating the involvement of people with aphasia in stroke research by developing communicatively accessible research resources. *Topics in Language Disorders, 37*(1), 67–84.

Popay, J. & Collins, M. (Eds) with the PiiAF Study Group (2014). *The Public Involvement Impact Assessment Framework Guidance.* UK: Universities of Lancaster, Liverpool and Exeter.

Rose, T.A., Worrall, L.E., Hickson, L.M., & Hoffmann, T.C. (2011). Aphasia friendly written health information: Content and design characteristics. *International Journal of Speech-Language Pathology, 13*(4), 335–347.

Volkmer, A. (Blog viewed January 2018) https://annavolkmersbigphdadventure.wordpress.com/2017/11/13/engaging-the-experts-in-every-which-way/

8 Evaluating training

Isla Jones

Introduction

The previous chapters have highlighted the need for training on and around the Mental Capacity Act (MCA, 2005) and how we can go about equipping our teams with the knowledge, skills and confidence to work to the highest standards in this area. But how do we evaluate the effectiveness of our training? In our busy, time-pressured days how do we know that the time spent training has been worthwhile? Pre- and post-training questionnaires are the most common evaluation tool in health settings (Cervai & Polo, 2015). Questionnaires are valuable for providing information about the participants' satisfaction with the training, and any 'new' knowledge gained. They do not, however, typically evaluate what knowledge has 'stuck' over time and, crucially perhaps, they do not reflect whether the new learning has been transferred into the workplace.

Knowledge is liable to decay unless used. Yet the transfer of new skills to daily use can be extremely tricky when faced with challenges such as competing work and clinical priorities, bureaucracy and organizational culture, to name but a few. Undoubtedly questionnaires have their place, but they need to be carefully designed and considered alongside other evaluation tools when thinking about how to best measure the effectiveness of training. Evaluating training is not simply a tick-box exercise; if we want to create change we need to know if our training is achieving its aims and how it can be improved. This chapter outlines some considerations when planning an evaluation and offers two models to assist in that planning. Evaluation tools are described and sample questions provided that can be used in your evaluations.

What to consider when planning your evaluation

It is important to plan your evaluation at the same time as planning your training. This ensures that your aims are measurable and that you allocate sufficient resources and time to the evaluation. Here are some considerations to help you choose or design the most appropriate evaluation tool(s) for your training session.

1. The aims of your training

Your training should be addressing an identified need. Therefore, your evaluation should be measuring if there has been a change in the specified area of need. Consider your aims and objectives carefully and make sure that they are measurable. This will assist you in thinking about what evaluation tools will work best to measure any change. Some examples of learning objectives might include:

- Trainees to feel more confident in carrying out capacity assessments
- Trainees to demonstrate understanding of the MCA including (define any key learning points)
- Trainees to demonstrate increased use of communication support tools in capacity assessments.

(More examples can be found in Table 2.6 of this book.)

2. Who will see your evaluation?

Nikols (2003) emphasizes that, although we may look for objective measures of training success, we must remember that judging whether the training has been of value is ultimately subjective; it is dependent on what matters to an individual. Clarifying what the recipients of your evaluation report want to see will assist you in defining the aims of the training, and thus selecting the evaluation tools that provide information of interest to your audience. So, for example, if you are carrying out a regular in-service as a 'refresher on the MCA', you (as the trainer) are likely to be the recipient of your evaluation. As such, you may want to pick a tool which is fast and easy to administer and that provides information on your training style, content and organization as well as measuring whether your aims have been met. Alternatively, if you have organized a day course for members of the multidisciplinary team (MDT) you are likely to want an array of measures that will assess whether your aims have been met, and provide information in a way that enables management to make decisions on future training.

3. What will the evaluation be used for?

A good evaluation ought to determine if the training should continue, enable improvements to the training, ensure learning has taken place, align the training with strategy, and demonstrate the value of the training (Kirkpatrick & Kirkpatrick,

2007). In the real world, it may not be possible or expedient to ensure that your evaluation is able to tick all of these boxes. Referring back to the previous example, if you are carrying out a regular in-service it might be less important that your evaluation rigorously demonstrates the value of your training, but more important that it enables you to develop your skills as a trainer. If you are carrying out a full day training session it may be more important to evaluate whether the time and money required to put on the training day has been justified by the training outcomes. Alternatively, you may want to use the evaluation as a means of determining a baseline level of knowledge, confidence or adherence to process, and continue to evaluate or audit these areas. Your evaluation could also be designed to form the basis for a piece of research. Determining the function of your evaluation is an essential consideration because the tools you use and questions you include will be driven not only by what you want to find out, but also by what you want to do with the information you obtain.

4. Time and resources

Thinking about your available time and resources is fundamental in enabling you to plan effectively. It may be that you have to make some difficult decisions about how much time you allocate to the training itself versus the evaluation. This is particularly pertinent if your intention is to carry out the evaluation during the training session. Obtaining well-considered answers requires time, resources and planning. It may be challenging to access trainees and to engage them in an evaluation after the event, but there is always the opportunity to be creative with available resources to maximize the possibility of completing a meaningful evaluation. For example, is there an assistant or even a volunteer who could interview trainees at times convenient to them? Could you use an online survey tool such as SurveyMonkey to disseminate feedback forms or questionnaires? Are you able to investigate some outcomes without directly involving the trainees? If one of your aims is to increase knowledge of organizational processes, could you audit some relevant case notes to determine if processes are being followed and if any change has occurred?

Think carefully about your own resources, including your skills, and be realistic about the time it takes to analyze any information you receive and to present it in a meaningful way. The evaluation will be meaningless unless the information is analyzed, received and genuinely understood by those who have an interest in addressing practice in mental capacity assessments and deciding whether the training should continue. Table 8.1 presents some questions that might assist you in considering your options.

Table 8.1 Questions to support you when planning your evaluation.

Evaluation planning considerations: Resource, skills and time	Trainer notes
What skills, time and resources do I have available to complete this evaluation?	
Estimate the time taken to gather evaluation information, analyze it and collate it into a report or presentation. How can I fit this into the allocated training time and my working week?	
How can I access my trainees after the training session and maximize the possibility of their engagement in my evaluation?	
Is there anybody who can assist me in carrying out my evaluations?	
How do I want my evaluation to be collated, analyzed and presented (detailed report, PowerPoint presentation, verbal presentation, list of four key discussion points). What time and resources will I need to complete this?	

Evaluation models

Knowing what to measure and subsequently what tools to use is not straightforward. As discussed above, you need to consider the recipients of the evaluation, the purpose of the evaluation and what judgements or decisions might be made based on your evaluation. It is also useful to look to the research literature in this area to consider what models of evaluation have been developed that can help. Two well-known training evaluation models are the Kirkpatrick Model of Evaluation (Kirkpatrick, 1967; Kirkpatrick & Kirkpatrick, 2007) and the Stakeholder Approach to Evaluating Training (Nickols, 2003).

Kirkpatrick Model of Evaluation

Although conceived some time ago, this model remains relevant in the training literature. It identifies four levels of evaluation. Each level builds on the previous one, and requires more rigorous and time-consuming analysis. The levels are:

1. **Reaction:** This is about trainees' perception of the training. Did they find it useful? How satisfied were they with the training? Did they like the way the information was delivered?

2. **Learning**: This could be learning in relation to knowledge, skills or attitudes. Do the trainees know more about the MCA and best interests' decision-making process as a result of the training? Have they developed new skills to help in carrying out capacity assessments?

3. **Behaviour**: Are the trainees using their new knowledge or skills? Is there an improvement in the way capacity assessments are being conducted? Is there evidence that the trainees' knowledge is affecting clinical decision making in applying the MCA process?

4. **Results**: Has the training met the need identified? This is usually about looking at the value of the training in terms that managers can appreciate. This might be as simple as demonstrating that all speech and language therapists (SLTs) are actively engaging in capacity assessments where appropriate, or that there is a reduction in the number of conflicts over capacity assessments within a multidisciplinary team, or that teams are using the appropriate documentation when completing capacity assessments.

Phillips (1997) added a fifth level to Kirkpatrick's model: 'Return on Investment'. This is the notion of determining the financial return on investment of training. It involves calculating or estimating the financial resources used to deliver the training versus the financial gains from having done so. This is not an easy task, and advice from managers used for calculating activity in current financial terms would be beneficial should be focusing on this.

The Kirkpatrick model is referenced widely in the training literature and indeed some health training studies have used it to good effect (Patterson et al., 2013). This study investigated the impact of simulation-based training on service user safety in a paediatric emergency department in America. The training involved techniques to prevent error and improve communication within the team. The training was delivered to groups of 8–10 multidisciplinary team members. At the start, the training took place over two days but eventually the programme was condensed to a four-hour session. Mini-lectures were delivered, videotapes and case studies reviewed, and simulations carried out with facilitated debriefs. The evaluation of the training included a satisfaction questionnaire (Level 1 of the Kirkpatrick model), a knowledge test (Level 2) and an evaluation of participant performance in the simulation but also on the ward (Level 3). The number of service user safety events were also gathered and compared to pre-training numbers (Level 4).

Although some studies have used the model successfully it is widely acknowledged that most training evaluation starts and ends at Level 1 of the

Kirkpatrick model. The reasons for this are not clear but there is the suggestion that perhaps the time taken to evaluate training at all of these levels outweighs the benefit of having done the training. For some it may be that this structure of evaluation does not inspire commitment from managers and those financing the evaluation. Nevertheless, it is worth considering Kirkpatrick's four levels of evaluation when making decisions about how to approach evaluation of training sessions.

Stakeholder approach to evaluating training

A more recent model is the 'Stakeholder approach to evaluating training' (Nickols, 2003). Nickols defines stakeholders as "a group or an individual with an interest in seeing a particular endeavour succeed". Specifically, stakeholders are defined as groups or individuals who 'put something in' to the training with an expectation of getting something out. This model may be more useful from a management perspective.

Nickols argues that what is most important to one stakeholder in a given training programme may be quite different from another stakeholder's requirements. So, for example, the trainees, as one stakeholder group, are likely to care primarily about the applicability of the training and the extent to which attending the session was worth the time out of their busy day. Alternatively, the manager releasing staff for the training might ultimately care about whether the training has reduced the time taken in supervision sessions to discuss capacity assessments.

Nickols' model suggests approaching the evaluation by:

• Identifying the key stakeholder groups
• Identifying the contributions and inducements (what they get out of the training) for each group
• Prioritizing these contributions and inducements and reducing them to a shortlist for each stakeholder
• Devising a simple way of measuring the satisfaction of the various stakeholders with their inducements
• Devising simple ways of measuring the value of the contribution made by various stakeholders.

He suggests incorporating this information into a stakeholder contributions-inducements score card. A simple example of a score card for an in-service is provided in Table 8.2.

If you wanted to use this model to plan your evaluation it would be

Table 8.2 Example score card for 30-minute in-service on the MCA.

Contribution	Stakeholder	Inducement
Time, attention, energy, knowledge, participation	Participant	Useful information and knowledge, tools, improved skills, improved status in work environment, professional development
Time, energy, skills, knowledge	Trainer	Recognition, personal satisfaction in accomplishment, new insight and knowledge, professional development
Resource commitments, support, leadership	SLT Manager	Improved job performance by employees, influence

important to speak with your stakeholders about their expected inducements rather than anticipating what these might be. In so doing this may help you to define the aims of your training and also to improve your ability to satisfy your stakeholders. If the score card is shared and discussed it should also encourage mutual accountability and responsibility for the success of the training.

Evaluation tools

Having determined the aims of your training, the audience and stakeholders, the time and resources available and the purpose of your evaluation you can then select the appropriate tool(s). Table 8.3 below lists some of the common tools used to evaluate training with their advantages and disadvantages.

Example tools

The following eight tables provide example questionnaires, rating scales, reflective observation questions, audit and observation checklists. These may be photocopied or integrated into your own bespoke evaluation tools. Consider using multiple choice questions or rating scales for quick analysis and open questions for more revealing answers.

> • All the following documents are available as free downloads at A4 size (with more space for answers) from the book's webpage at:
> http://www.jr-press.co.uk/speech-language-therapists-mental-capacity.html

Table 8.3 The advantages and disadvantages to different evaluation tools and how these might align with certain learning objectives.

Evaluation tool	Advantages	Disadvantages	Example learning objectives
Questionnaire (see examples in Table 8.4)	Quick to administer. If administered while trainees are in the room you are likely to get information from **everyone**. And has the advantage of maintaining a sense of anonymity; thus, trainees may provide a more honest response. You can make it easy to analyze by giving multiple choice options or rating scales or by using free software such as SurveyMonkey (SurveyMonkey. co.uk) which can collate responses and perform some basic analysis. Provides useful 'in the moment' information on the value of the training from the trainees' perspective and on the process of the training, e.g., room, content, trainer's style, etc.	Does not directly measure transfer of knowledge or skill to the workplace but, if administered sometime after the training, can be used to get stakeholder perspectives on whether knowledge or skills have been successfully transferred. Typically, this method does not provide space for in-depth information. This can be a disadvantage if you are wanting to explore why something worked or didn't work and the reasoning behind people's answers.	For trainees to understand the basic principles of the MCA. For trainees to understand the two-part assessment of mental capacity. For trainees to feel more confident in working with people on issues around decision making and mental capacity. For trainees to perceive the training to be valuable and enjoyable.
Rating scales (see example Table 8.4 & 8.9)	Can be used within questionnaires or interviews and is an easy and useful way to gain stakeholder opinions on whether their expectations have been met by the training and on their satisfaction, etc. The information provided is easy to analyze and report and can highlight key areas for change without too much work.	As with any quick and easy method it lacks depth and you are therefore unable to satisfactorily answer 'why' you got the results you did.	For trainees to feel more confident in working with people on issues around decision making and mental capacity. For trainees to perceive the training as valuable and/or enjoyable. For trainees to perceive the team as having a common understanding of issues around decision making and mental capacity.

Evaluation tool	Advantages	Disadvantages	Example learning objectives
Interviews	Interviewing the trainee about their experience of capacity assessments can get to the heart of where you want to see change.	Time-consuming both in administration and in analysis. In reality, you are unlikely to be able to interview all trainees so you may lose out on breadth of opinion what you will gain on depth of information.	For trainees to demonstrate an understanding of the impact of communication difficulties on mental capacity assessments.
	Enables your interviewee to provide more detail and thought-through responses. This can be particularly illuminating when you want to explore issues, perspectives and responses at a deeper level than that provided by a questionnaire.	Perceptions and opinion are very important but they may not be what most interests your audience. Consider what it is that your stakeholders are interested in and whether this is the best way to get information on what matters to them.	For trainees to carry out mental capacity assessments in accordance with the law and guidance provided by the MCA Code of Practice (2007).
	You can be flexible about where the interview takes place and when. If you choose to interview, consider asking the trainee for permission to record the interview as this will assist you when analyzing and creating your evaluation report.	Knowing how best to analyze and use qualitative data is a skill and you may require some guidance to make the most of your interview data. Thematic analysis can be effectively used to identify themes arising from the data (Braun & Clarke, 2006) but may require time and expertise to ensure it is rigorously applied.	For trainees to know when to refer to SLTs when considering issues of decision making and mental capacity for a particular individual.
	Interviews can be a useful way to explore whether trainees have used their new knowledge/skills and if not, why not.		For trainees to follow protocols and procedures in assessing communication and supporting service users with communication needs during a mental capacity assessment.
		People may say what they think you want to hear, rather than want they really think if you are interviewing them personally.	For trainees to feel confident in dealing with issues around decision-making and mental capacity.
			For trainees to understand and feel confident about what to do if there is conflict within the team about an individual's capacity to make a particular decision
Knowledge based test (see examples in Table 8.5 & 8.6)	Enables you to assess if any new learning has taken place and is an easy way to establish a baseline and knowledge-based learning objectives.	Can intimidate trainees and impact upon their attitude towards the training.	For trainees to demonstrate an understanding of the basic principles of the MCA.
	Easy to administer and to analyze, particularly if you are using multiple choice answers	Knowledge is rarely the end goal of training; how we use the knowledge is often more important. In today's work environments, we often have easy access to information on the intranet, in policies, and on the web, therefore a knowledge-based test should only form part of any training evaluation.	For trainees to demonstrate an understanding of the two-part assessment of mental capacity.
			For trainees to understand best-interest decision-making process.
			For trainees to understand and feel confident about what to do if there is conflict within the team about an individual's capacity to make a particular decision

(Continued over)

Evaluation tool	Advantages	Disadvantages	Example learning objectives
Case studies	A useful way to look at how trainees might transfer their new knowledge and skill without having to observe them 'on the job'. You can create specific case studies to ensure particular learning objectives are included (see Chapter 2 for examples). You can use case studies with appropriate question or problems to solve as pre- and post-tests to look at changes in problem solving and practice.	A response to a case study may not reflect what a person will do 'in real life'. You will need to consider carefully how you will analyze the responses and ensure that your case studies are likely to elicit the evidence of learning that you are looking for.	For trainees to be able to conduct an assessment of decision-making capacity selecting appropriate communication support tools. For trainees to understand the different roles an SLT may take when working with an individual who requires a mental capacity assessment. For trainees to feel more confident about carrying out mental capacity assessments. For trainees to engage in mental capacity assessments appropriately.
Observations (during training session simulations or i 'real life') (see Table 8.10 for example observation checklist)	The most direct way of assessing whether skills have been transferred into practice and the workplace.	Observing trainees may make them feel uncomfortable and cause a change in behaviour and dynamic between the trainee and trainer. You will need to get permission from all involved in the situation including the service user. You will need to create a careful observation checklist to ensure you can assess for learning and consider carrying out observations at the pre-training or at the beginning of the session and post-training or at the end of the session. This is a time-intensive exercise for the assessor, yet is more likely to result in carry over to practice than training alone. More subjective, and may be influenced by your presence; a trainee may perform differently when observed, additionally you may be more positively or negatively inclined to different people based on extraneous issues such as personality, etc.	For trainees to be able to conduct an assessment of decision-making capacity using communication support tools appropriately. For trainees to involve an SLT when appropriate in issues around decision making and mental capacity for a particular individual.

Evaluation tool	Advantages	Disadvantages	Example learning objectives
Case note audit (see Table 8.11 for example)	Enables analysis of practice without relying on cooperation of trainees once the training session has been completed.	The reliability of your findings is based upon the note writing practice of your organization and the trainees themselves. For example, a trainee may have increased their use of communication support tools but fail to record when they have used pen and paper or pictures in a particular capacity assessment. Dependent on access to notes this may be a relatively laborious task and you need to think carefully about how you will capture and present your findings.	For trainees to follow local capacity assessment protocols. For trainees to document capacity assessment rationale and findings using agreed proforma/ structure. Trainees to increase their use of supportive communication tools during capacity assessments and to document what they have used. Trainees to understand the value of a communication assessment prior to a capacity assessment where possible.
Activity measures (referral rates for capacity assessments, time spent on capacity assessments)	If this data is already collected by your team it may be a relatively easy way to look at the impact of your training on a measure that is meaningful to some stakeholders.	Beware any negative findings on these measures. There may be many reasons why referral rates have not increased despite an increase in trainee understanding of the SLT role. This could range from something as simple as understanding the referral process, to time pressure and politics. Using multiple evaluation methods is essential to ensure the wrong conclusions are not drawn and to elicit useful information.	Trainees to understand the role of speech therapists in decision-making capacity assessments and how to refer. Trainees to understand the key components of speech therapy intervention with regards to mental capacity.
Trainee self-report (in focus group, written reflection) (see examples in Tables 8.7 & 8.8)	Likely to provide depth of information. Active involvement of trainees in the evaluation process may encourage trainees to 'own' the learning and transfer knowledge and skills into the workplace. This method will not intimidate trainees in the way that observations might.	Time-consuming and relies on access to trainees and their willingness to provide time after the event. This may be subjective; people may not be entirely honest about their perceptions or what they are doing, or they may not have insight to how well they are doing things.	Increased participant confidence and (appropriate) involvement in capacity assessments. Improved understanding of the MCA and Code of Practice.

Table 8.4

Participant-focused questions
How relevant is the Mental Capacity Act (2005) to your day-to-day work?
Not at all relevant   Somewhat relevant   Highly relevant
In the area of mental capacity how motivated are you to change the way you work?
Not at all motivated   Somewhat motivated   Highly motivated
Please explain your answer:
Did you choose to attend this training? **Yes/no**
If no, please explain:
How confident do you feel about assessing decision-making capacity and following the Mental Capacity Act 2005 Code of Practice (2007)?
1   2   3   4   5
Not at all confident   Very confident
How confident do you feel in supporting people with communication difficulties during a capacity assessment?
1   2   3   4   5
Not at all confident   Very confident
How confident do you feel in supporting people around advance planning?
1   2   3   4   5
Not at all confident   Very confident
Do you feel comfortable supporting people who make unwise decisions? **Yes/no**
I know when to ask an SLT for support in assessing decision-making capacity.
Strongly disagree   Disagree   Unsure   Agree   Strongly agree
I think capacity assessments should be carried out by medical professionals only.
I agree   Disagree   Don't know
It should be possible to complete most capacity assessments in 10 minutes.
I agree   Disagree   Don't know
Capacity assessments do more harm than good.
I agree   Disagree   Don't know
Please explain your answer.
How would you rate the likelihood of conflict within your team about mental capacity assessments? Please circle the statement that most closely represents your view.
Never any conflict   Conflict is rare   Conflict occurs sometimes   Often there is conflict

Table 8.5

Knowledge-based questions for MDT or SLT trainees

1. A person with aphasia following a stroke has been assessed as not having capacity to make a decision about where they are going to live on discharge from hospital. This means (tick one response)

(a) They do not have capacity to make any decisions about health or social care

(b) They do not have capacity to make this particular decision at this particular time

2. The Mental Capacity Act (2005) is designed to… (pick one answer)

(a) Stop people making unwise decisions

(b) Assist and support people who might lack capacity and protect them from being overly restricted or controlled by other people

3. What areas does the Mental Capacity Act (2005) NOT cover (tick as many as you think are appropriate)

(a) Family relationships including marriage

(b) Voting rights

(c) Assisted suicide

d) Personal appearance

(e) Leisure activities

(f) Healthcare decisions

(g) Financial decisions

3. Circle the five key principles of the Mental Capacity Act (2005) from the following list

(a) A person must have a relative or representative present for a capacity assessment

(b) A person who refuses to engage in a capacity assessment must be deemed not to have capacity to make a particular decision

(c) A person must be assumed to have capacity unless it is established that he lacks capacity

(d) A person must have a capacity assessment if they make an unwise decision

(e) A person is not to be treated as unable to make a decision unless all practicable steps to help him to do so have been taken without success

(f) A person is not to be treated as unable to make a decision merely because he makes an unwise decision

(g) A decision made on behalf of a person who lacks capacity must be made in the presence of a family member or advocate for the person

(h) An act done, or decision made, under this Act for or on behalf of a person who lacks capacity must be done, or made, in his best interests.

(i) Before the act is done, or the decision is made, regard must be had to whether the purpose for which it is needed can be as effectively achieved in a way that is less restrictive of the person's rights and freedom of action.

(j) A person is not to be treated as unable to make a decision unless it is established he lacks capacity on three separate occasions

(Continued over)

4. How long does a person need to retain information relevant to the decision to be deemed to have capacity to make the decision in England/Scotland/NI?

(a) Over 24 hours

(b) Long enough to use it to make an effective decision

(c) Long enough to be able to act in accordance with the decision

5. An individual who lacks capacity should still be involved in the decision-making process (true/false)

6. Who can assess capacity (tick the correct answer)

(a) Only a psychiatrist or medical professional

(b) Any person depending on the nature of the decision

Table 8.6

Knowledge-based questions specifically for speech therapists
1. Your client's girlfriend tells you that before he had his head injury he had been very clear that he wanted to marry her and she would like to arrange this. Your client has no intelligible words and has an inconsistent yes/no response to complex questions. What do you do? (tick the most appropriate response/open written response)
(a) Assess the client's capacity to make a decision about marriage to his girlfriend. If he demonstrates that he does not have capacity to make this decision initiate a best interest process
(b) Assess the client's capacity to make a decision about marriage to his girlfriend. If he demonstrates that he does not have capacity to make this decision, explain to his girlfriend that the decision cannot be made for your client and therefore at present he would not be able to get married.
(c) Explain to your client's girlfriend that he does not have capacity to make the decision to get married based on what you know of his communication skills
(d) Refer to the Court of Protection
2. 'A person is not to be treated as unable to make a decision unless all practicable steps to help him to do so have been taken without success.' This is one of the core principles of the Mental Capacity Act (2005). What practical steps might you take to help a man with a learning disability, who is unable to read and write, to make a decision about surgery to remove his diabetic foot?

Table 8.7

Practice-based questions – Pre-training
1. What do you find challenging about decision-making capacity assessments?
2. When a capacity assessment is required, what do you find helpful in guiding your practice?
3. Are you actively involved in capacity assessments? If so, please briefly describe your role(s)
4. When would you involve an IMCA?
5. How do you know when a capacity assessment is required?
6. What do you typically do to prepare for a capacity assessment?

Table 8.8

Practice-based questions – Post-training
1. Since the training, what has changed in your work related to decision-making capacity assessments?
2. Can you recall three key points from the training that have influenced your current practice?
3. What barriers (if any) are there to using new knowledge or skills from the mental capacity training?
4. With hindsight what was useful about the training?

Table 8.9

Training-focused questions
1. How satisfied were you with the training session?
Not at all satisfied Slightly satisfied Neutral Moderately satisfied Very satisfied
Please explain your answer.
2. How satisfied were you with the content of the training session?
Not at all satisfied Slightly satisfied Neutral Moderately satisfied Very satisfied
Please explain your answer.
3. Were the aims of the training session clear? **Yes/No**
4. Was the training applicable to your work? **Yes/No**
5. What were two good things about the training and one thing you would like to see done differently or added
(1)
(2)
(3)
6. How satisfied were you with the facilities, room and materials?
Not at all satisfied   Slightly satisfied   Neutral   Moderately satisfied   Very satisfied
7. How satisfied were you with the delivery of the training?
Not at all satisfied   Slightly satisfied   Neutral   Moderately satisfied   Very satisfied

Table 8.10 Example observation checklist.

Observation	Yes	No	Comments
Information given to the person about the decision is: • accessible • relevant • targeted to the specific needs of the individual • sufficient to allow the person to make an informed choice about the specific decision in question • supported by tools such as visual aids, communication aids and hearing aids as appropriate (1.1.5)			
The practitioner is using information about the individual's wishes, beliefs and preferences to support decision making (1.1.6)			
Information provided complies with NHS Accessible Information Standards (1.2.6)			
Decision options are presented in a balanced and non-leading way (1.2.6)			
If the person has communication difficulties, strategies are used to support the person's understanding and support their ability to express themselves (1.2.9)			
Reasonable steps have been taken to ensure the assessment does not cause a person distress or harm (1.4.11)			

Observation checklist

This observation checklist (Table 8.10) is based on some of the guidance found in the draft NICE SICE Mental Capacity guidance (www.nice.org.uk/guidance/gid-ng10009/documents/draft-guideline). At the time of writing the full finalized guidelines have not been published. Consider creating your own chart to focus specifically on areas you have identified as needing improvement.

Audit form

This audit form (Table 8.11) uses some of the guidance found in the draft NICE SCIE Mental Capacity guidance, specifically items 1.2.17, 1.4.25, 1.4.26. The draft guidance can be found at www.nice.org.uk/guidance/gid-ng10009/

Table **8.11** Example audit form.

Audit item	Present in documentation	Missing in documentation	Comments
If the person has an impairment to their brain or mind			
Information given to the person			
Individuals involved in supporting the decision			
Steps taken to help the person make the decision			
Key considerations for the person in making the decision			
The decision reached			
Needs identified as a result of the decision			
Further actions arising from the decision			
If the person has capacity but makes an unwise decision			
If the person has capacity and gives valid consent			
Documented as a stand-alone assessment			

documents/draft-guideline. Recommendations on best interest meeting documentation has not been included but is incorporated in the draft NICE SCIE guidance section 1.5.

Conclusion

Planning your evaluation approach is as important as planning the training task itself. You will only get the information you ask for when evaluating capacity training activities. Therefore, consider carefully the tool(s) you decide to use and the questions you decide to ask. Ultimately, the information you glean from your evaluation should help you to maximize the impact of your training and create the change you are aiming for. To achieve this, you may need to trial different tools and questions to identify which best meet the needs of your audience, your commissioners, your managers and yourself.

A word of warning: there may be situations where you find that the change you were hoping to achieve has not occurred. If, for example, your evaluation has focused primarily on the trainees and their experience of the training session, you may know that they enjoyed the session and thought the content was relevant but you will not know why the transfer of knowledge or skills has not occurred. Or you might find concerns identified are more of a reflection of underlying organizational issues quite aside from the training you have delivered. Perhaps the barrier to changing practice is in fact the influence of a leading member of the team, or an existing departmental process that directly contradicts the information being presented. This will only be revealed by asking the right questions. Once the information is obtained, these barriers can be challenged. When planned carefully, your evaluation is a powerful tool that can influence change.

References

Braun, V. & Clarke, V. (2006). Using thematic analysis in psychology. *Qualitative Research in Psychology*, 3(2), 77-101.

Cervai, S. & Polo, F. (2015). Evaluating the quality of the learning outcome in healthcare sector: The Expero4care Model. *Journal of Workplace Learning*, 27(8), 611-626.

Kirkpatrick, D.L. (1967). Evaluation of training. In R.L. Craig & L.R. Bittel (Eds), *Training and Development Handbook* (pp. 87-112). New York: McGraw Hill.

Kirkpatrick, D.L. & Kirkpatrick, J.D. (2007) *Implementing the Four Levels: A Practical Guide for Effective Evaluation of Training Programs*. San Francisco: Berrett-Koehler Publishers.

Nickols, F. (2003). 'A stakeholder approach to evaluating training'. Accessed January 2018 at www.nickols.us/stakeholder.pdf

Patterson, M., Geis, G., LeMaster, T., & Wears, R. (2013). Impact of multidisciplinary simulation-based training on patient safety in a paediatric emergency department. *British Medical Journal Quality and Safety*, 22, 383-393.

Phillips, J. (1997). *Return on Investment in Training and Performance Improvement Programs*. Houston, TX: Gulf Publishing Company.

Index